Tai Chi
IN 10 WEEKS

Also by Dr. Aihan Kuhn

Natural Healing with Qigong
Simple Chinese Medicine
Tai Chi for Depression
Brain Fitness

Tai Chi
IN 10 WEEKS

Beginner's Guide

Dr. Aihan Kuhn
CMD, OBT

YMAA Publication Center
Wolfeboro, NH USA

YMAA Publication Center, Inc.
PO Box 480
Wolfeboro, New Hampshire, 03894
1-800-669-8892 • info@ymaa.com • www.ymaa.com

ISBN: 9781594395055 (print) • ISBN: 9781594395062 (ebook)

Edited by Doran Hunter and Leslie Takao
Cover design by Axie Breen
Photos by Ning Li
This book typeset in 12 pt. Adobe Garamond
Typesetting by Westchester Publishing Services

20200417

Publisher's Cataloging in Publication

Names: Kuhn, Aihan, author.
Title: Tai chi in 10 weeks : beginner's guide / Dr. Aihan Kuhn.
Description: Wolfeboro, NH, USA : YMAA Publication Center, Inc., [2017] | "A proven
  step-by-step plan to integrating the physical and psychological benefits of tai chi into
  your life." | Includes index.
Identifiers: ISBN: 9781594395055 (print) | 9781594395062 (ebook) | LCCN: 2017937191
Subjects: LCSH: Tai chi. | Tai chi—Health aspects. | Tai chi—Psychological aspects. |
  Qi (Chinese philosophy) | Body-mind centering. | Mind and body. | Physical fitness. |
  Self-care, Health. | Holistic medicine. | BISAC: SPORTS & RECREATION / Martial Arts &
  Self-Defense. | SCIENCE / Applied Sciences. | SPORTS & RECREATION / Training.
Classification: LCC: GV504 .K84 2017 | DDC: 613.7/148—dc23

Disclaimer

The practice, treatments, and methods described in this book should not be used as an alternative to professional medical diagnosis or treatment. The author and publisher of this book are NOT RESPONSIBLE in any manner whatsoever for any injury or negative effects that may occur through following the instructions and advice contained herein.

It is recommended that before beginning any treatment or exercise program you consult your medical professional to determine whether you should undertake this course of practice.

Editorial Notes

Romanization of Chinese Words

The interior of this book primarily uses the Pinyin romanization system of Chinese to English. In some instances, a more popular word may be used as an aid for reader convenience, such as "tai chi" in place of the Pinyin spelling, *taiji*. Pinyin is standard in the People's Republic of China and in several world organizations, including the United Nations. Pinyin, which was introduced in China in the 1950s, replaces the older Wade-Giles and Yale systems.

Some common conversions are found in the following:

Pinyin	Also spelled as	Pronunciation
qi	chi	chē
qigong	chi kung	chē gōng
qin na	chin na	chǐn nǎ
jin	jing	jǐn
gongfu	kung fu	gōng foo
taijiquan	tai chi chuan	tī jē chǔén

For more information, please refer to *The People's Republic of China: Administrative Atlas, The Reform of the Chinese Written Language,* or a contemporary manual of style.

Formats and Treatment of Chinese Words

The first instances of foreign words in the text proper are set in italics. Transliterations are provided frequently: for example, Eight Pieces of Brocade (Ba Duan Jin, 八段錦).

Chinese persons' names are mostly presented in their more popular English spelling. Capitalization is according to the *Chicago Manual of Style* 16th edition. The author or publisher may use a specific spelling or capitalization in respect to the living or deceased person. For example: Cheng, Man-ch'ing can be written as Zheng Manqing.

*I dedicate this book to my family,
my teachers, and my students.*

Contents

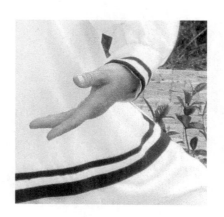

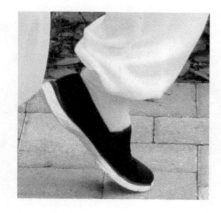

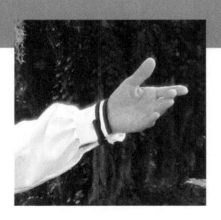

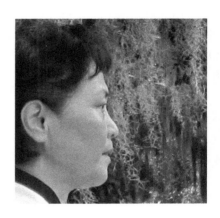

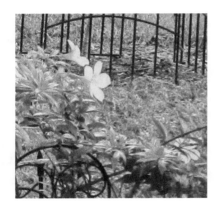

Preface

Welcome to the world of taiji (tai chi). As we will see, this is a timeless Chinese art with millions of practitioners all around the globe. Taiji has many facets. It is an art, as I have said, but it is also a type of meditation. It's an internal practice, a martial art, and a form of medicine. Taiji can be a social gathering and even exercise for brain fitness. I am excited to share this profound tradition with you.

When we practice taiji, we become part of a community that shares qi, or vital energy. Sharing qi creates a healing wave that is the key to well-being, peace, and happiness. This is a harmonious and healthy living group. Our community is growing stronger and bigger every year because we share qi. We give it and receive it from one another; it is endless and infinite. We help others with our qi.

When I was beginning my career as a doctor, my focus was mainly on treating disease. I empathized when I saw patients at the end stage of their illness and felt hopeless. I used to be sad when I saw patients suffering from an incurable illness, eventually dying. I realized there was nothing I could do.

Now my focus has changed. I have dedicated myself to prevention, holistic healing education, and helping people understand the importance of prevention. In this way, people can avoid getting a disease, or at least they have hope for healing. This work may not seem very impressive to some people, but it has tremendous value. I can help people avoid illnesses, bring back their happiness, prolong their lives, and help them increase the quality of their lives.

I enjoy being this kind of doctor—a doctor who cares about people's health, not only about disease. I believe this is what gives a doctor the most value.

My work has changed many lives. I've received several hundred letters from people I have treated and taught, and I can see and feel their happiness through their words.

Part of my success is from my patients and my students. They understand that prevention requires participation. They practice qigong and taiji on a regular basis, which is key to their healing. They are my heroes because they help themselves in the

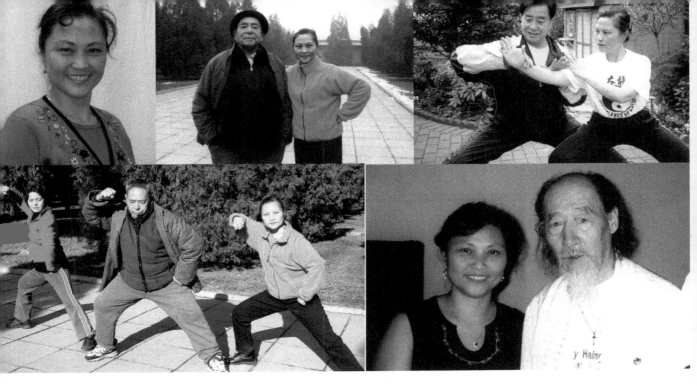

healing process, and they encourage me to continue my work. This is the work of a lifetime, just as taiji is a lifetime pursuit.

That brings us to the title of this book: *Tai Chi in 10 Weeks*. Can you really learn taiji in ten weeks? You cannot become a taiji master, of course, but you can learn the fundamentals of this art. You can build the foundation for this life-changing journey.

As a starting place, you will need to read the whole book. I suggest you use a pencil or pen to mark sections you think will be important for future review. Review your notes after you have been practicing taiji for six months. Studying in this way will help you to better understand this art, and you will be able to learn relatively fast. Regular practice is very important if you want to truly understand the nature of taiji and qigong. The theory and practice of taiji and qigong go hand in hand and stand side by side; one is not more important than the other.

In order to gain maximum benefits from practice, I recommend that students and instructors follow the taiji principles and pursue a structured learning experience, which can speed up the learning process. This book is intended to help students, instructors, and practitioners understand taiji theory and technique, as well as help them to have a better experience with learning and practicing, both in a group and as individuals.

If you want to use taiji for healing chronic issues, this book not only helps you understand how to do that but also guides you through the routine. You will find your self-study and practice easy and enjoyable.

If you are an instructor, this book will help you become more confident and more knowledgeable so your teaching may attract more students. You will be able to answer students' questions and instruct students at different levels.

The book is presented in a straightforward and organized fashion. The easy-to-read chapters and useful illustrations make learning simple and fun. Once you have read through the book once or twice, you will have a very good understanding of the approach to taiji study and the philosophy that goes with it.

You can use this book to supplement any classes or video instruction on the twenty-four-step form. I also invite you to try the companion DVD, *Tai Chi in 10 Weeks* (YMAA, 2017).

Being involved in taiji and qigong exercise is a wonderful learning and healing journey. People from all over the world practice these arts for their health and healing benefits. These benefits include improving internal and external strength, refining internal harmony, restoring mental clarity, balancing emotions, and developing better overall health. Additionally, people can enjoy the sensation and satisfaction that come from practicing taiji and qigong. As you practice for a while, you become more and more familiar with your own energy, your passion, and your feelings. You also improve your intuition, which helps you identify the positive and negative influences in your life. You can see what flows and what does not flow, and your enhanced intuition will ultimately guide you to go with the flow. Going with the flow not only reduces your stress but also helps you continue to move forward in life.

No one can live forever, but everyone can find ways to enjoy good health, happiness, and however much time we may have ahead. If we have many physical illnesses and struggle on a daily basis, or if we struggle with our mental and emotional issues, we lose the precious time we have. That is not quality living.

Taiji and qigong have already changed my life in many ways. It is the science of *energy medicine* that Western scientists have just begun paying attention to.

I wish you a wonderful journey of healing in taiji and qigong.

Dr. Aihan Kuhn

Moral Qualities of the Taiji Student

(Twelve Commitments)

1. The taiji student will not be prejudiced, judgmental, or biased regarding anyone's economic position, religion, race, or health condition. The taiji student will be accepting of people of all races, all abilities, and all ages as a part of the taiji family. The taiji student is kind to people.

2. The taiji student respects masters, instructors, and students at all levels.

3. The taiji student respects the practice facility and takes care of the facility, just as if it were his or her own house.

4. The taiji student shares knowledge and experience with others, helps others, and has only good intentions.

5. The taiji student will study taiji with modesty and practice diligently.

6. The taiji student is sincere and honest with himself or herself and with others.

7. The taiji student forgives others on all occasions.

8. The taiji student obeys all the rules of the school.

9. The taiji student understands and respects Daoist philosophy. The taiji student does not hate, hold grudges, or hold on to negative energy.

10. The taiji student loves and cares about his or her own person, just as he or she loves and cares about others.

11. The taiji student cherishes group energy and friendship.

12. The taiji student will only use the taiji martial skill for the protection of self, family, and other people in an urgent situation, never intending to show off.

CHAPTER 1

What Is Taiji?

TAIJI IS AN ANCIENT CHINESE EXERCISE for health improvement, spiritual growth, disease prevention, healing assistance, and self-defense. It involves slow, circular movements; mental concentration; breath control; relaxation; and meditation. It has been proven that the practice of taiji offers great health benefits, including improvements in circulation, metabolism, balance, flexibility, posture, mental focus, immune function, daily energy levels, organ function, emotional balance, self-awareness, and brain health. Taiji is an exercise for all ages and all fitness levels. It is a sophisticated form of exercise that works on internal energy and manifests externally. It is a gift from the Chinese culture.

Taiji is the abridged name of taijiquan. "Tai" in Chinese means "bigger than big," "ji" means "extreme," and "quan" means "boxing." Taiji used to be called "soft boxing." Altogether, taijiquan can be translated as "grand force boxing." Taiji's focus is on inner energy and achieving inner peace through movement.

Taiji has many qualities. It is a form of *art* that can be observed in its beautiful movements. It intrigues people from all over the world. When you watch people in the park doing taiji, you may feel like they are performing a slow, graceful, fluid dance. You can feel the harmony in the taiji form, but you don't see the power in those graceful movements. There is an ancient Chinese proverb by Sun Tzu, the author of *The Art of War*: "to win without fighting."

Taiji is a form of *meditation*. It is sometimes called moving meditation or walking meditation. This kind of meditation helps you detach from stress in daily life and allows you to move on and move forward. In addition to stress relief, practicing this meditation also helps you balance your emotions and removes much of the mental "junk" that accumulates in our lives. By "junk" I mean useless thoughts or thoughts that make you unhappy. Some people practice sitting meditation, and others like moving meditation. Both are good; it just depends on how you like to meditate. For people

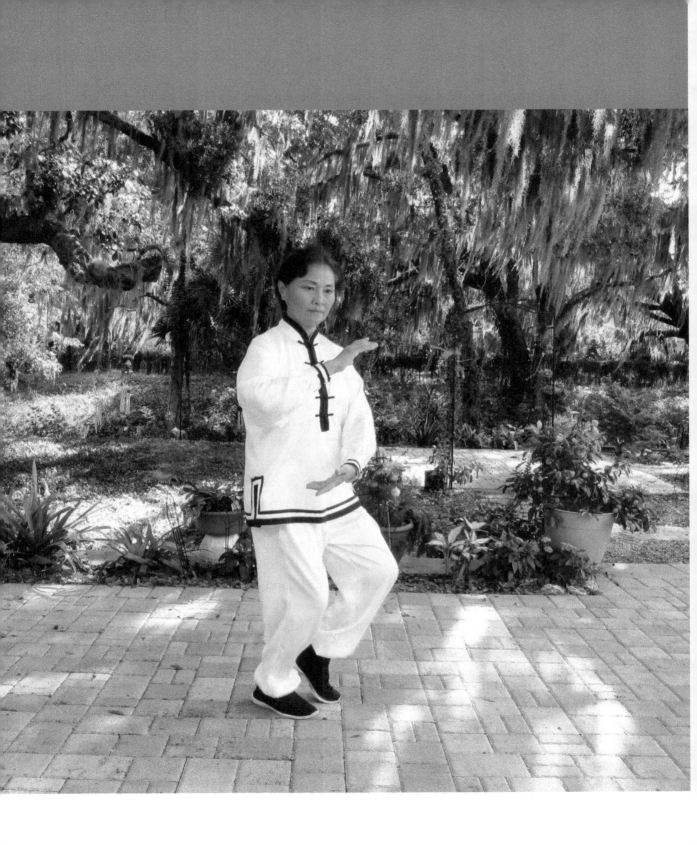

who have arthritis, fibromyalgia, or other circulation problems, taiji and qigong are much better than sitting meditation.

Taiji is an *internal practice* that builds your strength internally and externally. Taiji is a type of qigong; it is considered the higher level of qigong. Qigong is also an internal practice. In general, qigong is simpler and easier than taiji. Taiji movements are much more difficult, and you will need time to learn and practice.

Taiji is a *martial art*. In every movement of taiji, you can find a martial arts application that can be used for self-defense. As you practice and proceed to higher levels, you will understand its martial aspect and martial application. Taiji "push hands" is to practice taiji martial skill or taiji martial application. In taiji push hands, we say, "Four ounces can defeat a thousand pounds." In other words, taiji has power if applied.

Taiji and qigong are often called *energy medicine* or *preventive medicine*. The term "energy medicine" can be confusing; it has many meanings. In taiji we refer to a real internal energy workout that improves your qi, your vital energy. You can see and feel the results. Through qi practice, your self-healing ability and your immune system both improve. Not only can you heal yourself, but you can also prevent sickness and plateauing in life. In many cases, taiji and qigong can assist in the treatment and healing of chronic illnesses. From my own experience, taiji and qigong have helped with many of my ailments: asthma, arthritis, aches, pains, and negative emotions. It has also made me stronger internally. For people with cancer, both taiji and qigong can be excellent natural healing methods for enhancing organ and immune system function, which is the key to fighting cancer.

Taiji can be a type of *social gathering*—a "qi group." Taiji can be a group energy workout. The group practice creates a "qi field." The qi field affects individuals in a nurturing and positive way. That is why you feel good every time you practice in a group, even if you do not totally understand taiji or if you have not been doing taiji for long. This does not mean you must practice with other people every time. You still get benefits if you practice by yourself. When you reach a higher level, practicing taiji by yourself can really help you work on your qi, develop your concentration, improve your internal condition, and be grounded.

Taiji is a special type of *brain fitness practice*. Taiji and qigong can quiet your mind and regulate your breath. Regulating your breath not only allows your brain to rest but also brings more oxygen to the body and brain through deep breathing. In addition, the special movements of taiji stimulate and activate all parts of the brain. This is why people who practice taiji regularly show well-rounded living skills: balanced emotions, intuition, cognitive function, problem-solving skills, ability to learn quickly, logical decision making, and organization. In my book *Brain Fitness*, I describe in more detail how taiji affects our brains.

The benefits of practicing taiji and qigong are phenomenal. It benefits the entire body from head to toe. It strengthens muscles, tendons, joints, and circulation of blood and energy. It improves the immune system, mental concentration, balance, coordination, alertness, learning ability, and much more. As you start to explore the path of taiji, you will discover many other benefits too.

Mind-Body-Spirit

Eastern exercises always emphasize wholeness—the mind, the body, and the spirit. By contrast, most Western-style exercises are mainly focused on developing the body.

Why are our mind, body, and spirit important?

Our *mind* is the thinking part of our existence and determines how we walk, how we read and analyze data, how we communicate, how we make decisions, and how we solve problems. The *body* is the physical part of our existence, doing the eating, sleeping, walking, jogging, cooking, using tools, driving, and other physiological activities. The *spirit* is the meaningful part of our existence. It is where our hopes, our dreams, our beliefs, our passions, our fears, our love, and our hate are expressed. All of these parts are equally important. Taiji has the potential to bridge these parts by putting the practitioner in a state of mind where the connections among them are clear. When the three parts are in harmony, our body is strong, our mind is clear, and our spirit is pure and superior. This is what we call reaching the peak of qi.

Taiji touches all aspects of the person at the same time, reinforcing the perception that these so-called separate parts are but different aspects of the whole person. Taiji helps to open the body's energy pathways when practiced with mind, body, and spirit. It is not enough to simply copy the physical movements. By practicing taiji, you must incorporate all three parts through relaxation, meditation, concentration, study of ancient texts, and taiji theory.

Jing-Qi-Shen

In Chinese medicine, there are three fundamental substances called *jing*, *qi*, and *shen*. They are close in meaning to our Western terms *body*, *mind*, and *spirit*. These fundamental substances work side by side to keep us healthy.

Jing is usually translated as "original essence" and has a very close relationship to the Western term *gene*, or *genetic material*. Jing is stored in the kidneys. It is crucial to the development of the individual throughout life. Inherited at birth, jing allows us to develop from childhood to adulthood and then to old age. It governs growth, reproduction, and development; promotes kidney qi; and works with qi to help protect the body from external pathogens. Any developmental disorder such as learning difficulties or physical disabilities in children may be due to a deficiency of jing from birth. Other disorders such as infertility, poor memory, a tendency to get sick or catch colds, and allergies may also be due to deficiency of jing.

Qi refers to vital energy or life-force flow in the body. It is like the electric currents moving through a wire. There are various types of qi in the body working together to keep the physical and mental parts of our body in harmony. Qi has a very close relationship to human metabolism, immune function, digestion, absorption, emotion, breathing, mental clarity, and more. Qi is present internally and externally and controls the function of all parts of the body. Qi is like the motor in a car. Qi keeps us moving and functioning, keeps us warm, and protects us against sickness. Everything we do involves qi. Walking, eating, laughing, crying, playing sports, working, hiking, and writing are all related to qi. Qi affects our life every day. We cannot see the qi in the body, but we can feel it. We can feel when our energy is low and when it is high. We can sense if we are optimistic or depressed, if we are negative or positive; we can feel if our bodies are out of balance. Qi affects our health mentally, physically, and emotionally.

Shen refers to our spiritual energy, our highest consciousness, our connection with universal energies. Shen can also mean mental strength.

The English word *spirit* has many different meanings and connotations but commonly refers to a supernatural being or essence that is transcendent and therefore metaphysical. The *Concise Oxford English Dictionary* defines it as "the non-physical part of a person." For many people, however, spirit, like soul, forms a natural part of a being, not a transcendent one. Such people may identify spirit with mind or with consciousness or with the brain. But in Chinese, shen is more than just the mind. You can have lots of mental activity but lack shen; conversely, you can have excellent shen but have less mental activity because shen can make you focused.

Some people refer to shen as a soul. But in Chinese medicine theory, shen and soul are two different things though with some similarities. Soul is the immaterial or eternal part of a living being, commonly held to be separable from the body. Shen in traditional Chinese medicine (TCM) is the higher or energized eternal part of a living being.

Jing, qi, and shen are built on one another. Proficient jing leads to balanced qi. Balanced qi creates better shen. Improving the circulation of qi enhances and strengthens jing, as well as lifting shen. Good shen can control and connect to qi and be a guide to create more balanced qi. The cycle goes on and on, each substance affecting the others in both positive and negative ways.

By practicing taiji and qigong, you can strengthen the storage of jing, smooth the flow of qi, and build better shen. You can improve physical health, psychological well-being, and expand and enhance the spirit.

I have been teaching taiji and qigong for more than thirty years. I have seen students succeed in decreasing their stress level, improving physical strength, balancing their emotions, and increasing their overall health. They have gained in flexibility, stamina, balance, poise, skill in interpersonal interactions, and mental focus.

TAIJI IS NOT JUST FOR SENIOR CITIZENS; IT IS FOR EVERYONE

A common misconception is that taiji is only for old people. Because seniors are limited in many physical exercises, and taiji and qigong movements are slow, gentle, and low impact, it is ideally suited for seniors. But this does not mean it is only for the older generation. Taiji is for everyone, even for younger people. Oftentimes, I hear my students say, "I wish the kids would learn taiji." When I had my taiji school in Massachusetts, I had one class called Taiji for Kids. This is a special form of taiji designed for children. After each ten-week session, I saw many improvements in these children: better communication, better discipline, better flexibility, better manners, and improved academics. Two kids with Asperger's syndrome had dramatically improved their social and emotional skills. This supports the theory that taiji can have a great impact on our brains and change our lives.

It is not necessary for senior citizens to do the movements completely correctly as long as they can move their bodies and go with the flow of the form. By doing the movements, they can gain benefits. Daily practice of taiji not only helps senior citizens minimize physical discomfort but also helps them prevent illnesses and delays the aging process. For young people, taiji helps build a strong body and mind, increases the ability to focus, as well as helps to prevent disease.

Some people tell me that taiji seems too slow and doesn't look like a physical work-out. Taiji is largely internal. That is why most people don't choose taiji for their physical exercise. This is fine. Taiji is not for everyone even though taiji's health benefits make it an above-average exercise. People are attracted to different exercises, philosophies, food, and activities. The more people share their stories about practicing taiji and qigong, the more people will join this practice. The reality is that taiji is subtle and slow, but it is very powerful.

In our fast-paced society, we need slow and balanced exercise to help regulate our lives. Being busy all the time is stressful to the mind and abusive to the body. Eventually, the body breaks down. We all know that stress is the number one cause of disease. If the stress hormones adrenaline and noradrenaline are elevated for a long time, our heart is overstimulated and exhausted; then suddenly, we have heart disease. It happens to other organs too. Stress-related diseases of the body include, but are not limited to, fibromyalgia, hypertension, gastritis, diabetes, pneumonia, and breast cancer.

Life span depends on many things, such as stress, hygiene, medical condition, economic status, and education about prevention. In certain areas of Japan where people live in harmony with minimum stress, the average life span is much longer. People who practice taiji and qigong also live longer.

Most people who practice external martial arts when they are young eventually change to practice taiji (internal martial art) or qigong when they are older. As you get older, the external martial arts do more harm than good, but internal martial arts only benefit you. And even though taiji is an internal martial art, it perfects the external martial art as well as strengthens it.

The Benefits of Taiji in Four Major Parts

Physical

Taiji enhances physical stamina and strength. It balances the immune system, harmonizes and strengthens the organ systems, and increases metabolism. Students often say to me that they are stronger in general and also some even lost weight. Many students mentioned they are less sick during winter when other people get colds or upper respiratory infections. From teaching taiji for more than thirty years, I have seen many changes in students' health—even their chronic issues have improved. It is especially satisfying when I hear positive things from senior citizens. Some of them even reduced their medication because of the increase in the quality of their lives. In general, when age increases, health decreases. But with taiji and qigong practice, your health is maintained; this is the reason we call it preventive medicine.

Taiji has numerous, scientifically verified health benefits. A 2006 study published in *Alternative Therapies in Health and Medicine* reported great improvements in both lower-body and upper-body strength for older adults who began practicing taiji and were previously of a below-average fitness level and had at least one cardiovascular risk factor. The same study showed improvements in strength and flexibility for women in particular. A major Japanese study confirmed the results for strength and showed improvements as good as resistance training and even better than brisk walking.

Other studies demonstrate that taiji improves balance and reduces falls. This may be due to taiji's ability to enhance proprioception, the ability to sense one's own body in space. Taiji has been shown to significantly offset the decline in this ability, which comes with age. Also interesting is that just being afraid of falling makes you more likely to fall, and taiji helps reduce this fear. In addition to these benefits, taiji has shown great promise in helping with other conditions such as arthritis, low bone density, breast cancer, heart disease, high blood pressure, Parkinson's disease, sleep problems, and stroke.[1]

Mental

Practicing or learning taiji makes you calm and less stressed. In my book *Tai Chi for Depression*, I explain clearly how this balances human emotion through brain stimulation from specially choreographed body movements. People who practice taiji for a lifetime rarely have mental issues and tend to make the most out of life. If something dramatic happens, they can handle it with the right attitude.

The antiaging benefits of taiji practice give you mental clarity, improving your logical thinking and ability to do things in an efficient way. Your creativity is awakened, which can make your life more fun and enjoyable. Your renewed alertness helps you keep relationships and friendships strong. You maintain memory or sometimes even increase your memory.

Emotional

People who practice taiji seriously tend to have better control of their emotions, displaying an evenness of mood and a tendency to stay calm and peaceful. They are able to better control their emotions when stress or conflict arise and are able to let things go more easily. This is because of the smooth energy flow in their body, which also flows to the brain. There will be more details on this in chapter 2, "How Taiji and Qigong Prevent Brain Aging and Memory Loss."

Spiritual

The spirit is that which is beyond the ordinary. It is an intangible, higher consciousness that never dies. It connects us with ourselves, both physically and emotionally. Spirit defines who we are, how we think, what we think, and how we relate to the universe. It also describes both how we view God and our relationship with God. Spirit is a special energy that cannot be seen, heard, touched, or otherwise experienced materially. It can, however, be felt or experienced internally by ourselves, by people around us, and even by animals. My son has a dog I used to take care of. She is a lovely dog and extremely special. When my spirit energy is poor, she can sense it. She comes to sit near me and tries to be very quiet. When my spirit energy is high, she wants to play. Fortunately, my spirit energy is usually pretty good. But I cannot play all the time. Our spirits are on a constant path toward enlightenment, always weighing, experiencing, and reacting to life's yin (receptive, dark, feminine) and yang (active, bright, masculine) sides.

The meditation aspect of taiji allows us to tap into and activate our spirits. Our mind translates what our body feels as we move, and it interprets our spirits at the same time. Blended into the movement, our mind melts into the atmosphere of nature, beyond explanation. Therefore, we say taiji is an expression of spirit by way of the mind and body. When we practice as a group, our spirits coalesce. The group energy magnifies and we then express in unity, or as one. Whether we practice taiji alone or with others, we are connecting body, mind, and spirit with the whole universe.

Unlike meditation, practicing taiji cultivates the energy and the spirit, as well as balancing our own yin and yang. It allows us not to be absorbed or overtaken by negative spirit, or negative energy. It is as though taiji helps us to create a shield against negative energy. We tend to gravitate more toward people with positive spirit and energy, and we easily embrace positive spirit and energy.

Mind, body, and spirit connect with one another and affect one another in positive and negative ways. When your mind, body, and spirit are in harmony, you appear at peace with yourself. You become aware of your energy and feel the effects of taiji in your body. Additionally, you enjoy the sensation of satisfaction that comes from performing the movements. This is a journey that may not be easy, but it is very rewarding, especially as the benefits are manifested in later life.

Taiji has already changed my life in numerous ways. It is as much of an energy medicine for me as it is for other people. It is an energy medicine science, which Western scientists are finally starting to recognize. The best way of learning this true art of healing and well-being is by experiencing it. To find out how much you can get from taiji practice, start your journey today.

DAOIST PRACTICE

Taiji, qigong, and Chinese medicine all come from Daoist (Taoist) practice. In Daoist philosophy, everything on earth has two opposite sides: yin and yang. In order to keep the balance of the cosmos, it is important to keep the balance of the yin and the yang. In times of tragedy, chaos, and instability, as well as in cases of health problems, we often see an imbalance of yin and yang. When practicing taiji, you are following the Daoist practice that helps you to be more relaxed, be more balanced, let go of things more easily, and keep an inner peace. There are many translations of *Tao Te Ching* (also spelled *Daodejing*) in bookstores. I recommend that you find any copy and read a chapter a day. When you do so, you will realize how much wisdom it contains and how realistic and practical it is.

Taiji is a life journey. The sophisticated movements of taiji provide you with an endless learning experience that benefits both body and mind. Every year you gain multiple benefits physically, mentally, emotionally, and spiritually. A brief study of taiji does not mean you have learned taiji; it only means you have had a little taste of it. If you don't have a good instructor, you may not even be able to say that you had a little taste of it. Just learning a taiji form is not enough; you must practice the art fully, and practice regularly, to truly enjoy the benefits.

When you practice taiji consistently, you are a special person because not everyone has the patience or discipline for the long journey. Olympic athletes work very hard, year after year to get their medals. Similarly, as a taiji practitioner, you work hard year after year to get the "medal of a better life," a "medal of good health," and a "medal of a special person." The medals from taiji practice bring you a lifetime of satisfaction. Such satisfaction can help you to excel in whatever you do. This medal is invisible, but its value is immeasurable.

CHAPTER 2

How Taiji and Qigong Work in Human Healing

IN THE NATURAL HEALING SYSTEM, your mind and your body should not be separated. Your body can affect your mind, and your mind can affect your body. The energy pathways that go through your body also go through your brain and affect all parts of it, including neurochemicals.

Both taiji and qigong work with internal energy that brings harmony to the organ system. A harmonious organ system helps balance the body's biochemistry, hormones, and metabolism. This is how your healing ability becomes enhanced. When you have surgery, your wound may be healed in days or weeks, even months. It all depends on your level of healing ability. When you catch a cold, you may recover in days, weeks, or months; this also depends on your healing ability. If your healing ability is strong, you can heal any illness. Some people don't believe this, especially medical people. I was one of them, believing in what we studied in medical school and nothing else. I was trained in conventional medicine and believed it is always right. However, the past thirty years of experience has changed my view. I am now advocating natural medicine, natural healing, and preventive medicine. Think for a moment with your own common sense: when you are stressed for a long time, your body parts start to have problems, right? Your problem is less likely to be healed, or it takes much too long to heal, which means your healing ability is poor or weak. The power of taiji and qigong to improve your healing ability is a compelling reason to get started on your taiji journey. Here is how taiji and qigong are associated with healing.

The Body Meridians

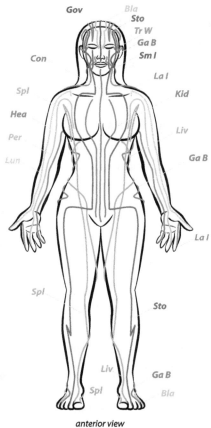

Gov
Bla
Sto
Tr W
Ga B
Sm I
Con
La I
Spl
Kid
Hea
Liv
Per
Lun
Ga B
La I
Spl
Sto
Liv
Ga B
Spl
Bla

anterior view

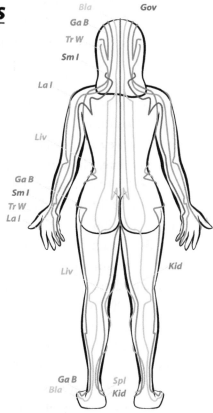

Bla
Gov
Ga B
Tr W
Sm I
La I
Liv
Ga B
Sm I
Tr W
La I
Liv
Kid
Ga B
Spl
Bla
Kid

posterior view

Two Centerline Meridians:

Conception Vessel
Governing Vessel

Twelve Principal Meridians:

Stomach Meridian
Spleen Meridian

Small Intestine Meridian
Heart Meridian

Bladder Meridian
Kidney Meridian

Pericardium Meridian
Triple Warmer Meridian

Gall Bladder Meridian
Liver Meridian

Lung Meridian
Large Intestine Meridian

Health Benefits of Taiji and Qigong

Cardiovascular Support

The slow and meditative movements of taiji and qigong improve function of the vagus nerve, also called the parasympathetic nerve, which is part of the autonomic nervous system. In the human body, all functions are controlled through the nervous system, and all organs and glands are controlled through the autonomic nervous system. The autonomic nervous system has two parts: the sympathetic function and the parasympathetic function. They are relatively opposite in what they do. For example, the sympathetic nerve causes an artery to contract while the parasympathetic nerve causes an artery to dilate. The sympathetic division is at work in action requiring a quick response, such as "fight or flight," and the parasympathetic division is involved in actions that do not require immediate action, such as "rest and digest," These two systems regulate and modulate vital functions in a usually antagonistic fashion to achieve homeostasis.

Taiji practice activates the parasympathetic function so that the heart rate and blood pressure are reduced, digestive function is improved, and the heart itself is rested and nourished by qi and blood.

In 1990, I went to China for the first time after moving to America. I got up in the morning the day after I arrived to walk the streets and try to reconnect with the place I once called home. I saw a bunch of seniors doing qigong on the street in an open spot. I studied this form of qigong when I was living in China so I knew it very well. I walked to the last row of people and joined their practice. After the group practice, I had a conversation with the woman next to me. She said she had had several heart attacks before and went to the emergency room every time. After practicing qigong for a year, she didn't need to go to the hospital. Her heart was normal again after practicing qigong daily for a year. She comes to the morning practice every day, rain or shine, on hot days and cold days—she never misses it. Inspired by her story, I brought this qigong form to the United States. This is the form I teach in my qigong instructor-training course called Therapeutic Qigong.

Respiratory Support

One of the most obvious elements of taiji and qigong practice is the breath. Both taiji and qigong require controlled, deep breathing. From deep breathing, our body gets more oxygen, and our respiratory system is well exercised. This concept is relatively easier to understand than the deep breathing that increases oxygen levels in the blood, organ system, and brain. The human body needs oxygen to survive and to heal. In our stressful world, we very often forget how to breathe—our breath is shallow. We wonder why we yawn so much during working hours. The reason is our brain's lack of oxygen. Even if we just take five deep breaths every hour, we feel the difference: more alert, awake, clear minded. The more oxygen you bring into the body, the better you feel.

Taiji and qigong not only increase the oxygen flow in the body but also increases its usage by organs and tissue. That is why taiji and qigong are considered natural antioxidants. This helps delay the aging process as well. In addition, taiji and qigong exercises improve lung energy and boost the immune system, which helps prevent respiratory infection, cold, flu, or any kind of lung disease. In Chinese medicine, lung energy is defensive energy that is related to the immune system in the respiratory track. By improving lung energy, the respiratory defense system improves. Therefore, there is less chance of catching a cold, flu, or other respiratory infection if we practice regularly.

Gastrointestinal Support

Taiji and qigong improve the autonomic nervous system, including both the sympathetic nervous system and the parasympathetic nervous system. Later in this chapter, you will find more information about the autonomic nervous system and how it relates to our health. When the parasympathetic nerve function is activated, the benefits show especially in the digestive organs because it promotes digestion and absorption. The mobility of the digestive track along with digestive enzymes and other digestive chemicals are more likely to stay at healthy levels. If mobility of the digestive track is normal, you have normal elimination. We call this natural cleansing and detoxification. You know you don't feel well if you cannot go to the bathroom for several days.

When your digestive function is normal, the food you eat will be properly used and transformed to energy. Otherwise, the food you eat will not be transformed to energy and you may feel tired even though you eat healthily. Some qigong forms involve self-massage of your abdominals and meridians, which is very beneficial to digestive organs. I was surprised to see so many cases of digestive illness in the United States. I have many patients with digestive illnesses and find relief through practicing taiji and qigong. In some cases I have to treat patients with natural remedies and natural methodologies. I always see better results from those who incorporate qigong into their therapy.

Many people use supplements. There is nothing wrong with this; we all need some nutritional support, especially during the aging or healing processes. Supplements can help you if your digestive system functions well and is able to absorb the nutrients. If you have an imbalance in the digestive system, however, using supplements is rather wasteful because they are not efficiently absorbed to be used for your needs. True masters or practitioners of taiji and qigong rarely have digestive problems, not only because they eat healthily but also because they practice their healing art diligently.

Musculoskeletal Support

Taiji and qigong involve whole-body, multidimensional movements with flexion, contraction, stretching, and strengthening. Your muscles get well-balanced exercise during taiji. This is also true with the therapeutic qigong course I teach. Your muscles and joints are in constant motion and receive plenty of oxygen from deep breathing. This not only keeps you fit but also keeps your muscles and joints healthy. You will have less muscle tension and stiffness. This helps delay aging of your muscles and joints, prevents degeneration, and maintains good muscle resiliency and flexibility. Healthy muscles and tendons can also prevent arthritis, fibromyalgia, and tendonitis. You will feel younger overall, with fewer aches and pains and less stiffness.

One of my students told me that she had fibromyalgia for many years. She went to her doctor to find answers, and her doctor said there is no cure, only pain medication. After she took my training, she practiced diligently and noticed her pain had reduced 90 percent. She could not be happier and felt it was a true lifesaver. When she had pain, she was depressed, struggled every day, and had low quality of life. She can now enjoy every part of life like other people.

Increase Stamina, Daily Energy Levels, and Immune Function

People who practice taiji not only improve their balance and coordination but also their immunity. A study from the Neuropsychiatric Institute at the University of California, Los Angeles[2], showed very interesting results in a group of older men and women who practiced taiji for forty-five minutes, three days a week. They showed an increase of up to 50 percent of memory T-cells. These are the immune system cells that identify and fight the varicella herpes virus, which causes shingles. People who have had chicken pox are vulnerable to shingles because the virus can remain dormant in nerve cells indefinitely. As we get older our immune system gets weaker, so the virus can wake up. Then you may have the symptoms of shingles, which causes blisters on the skin and is very painful.

Many people have told me how much they have improved their energy. Many have also told me they are lucky to be able to avoid sickness even though people around them get sick. They are able to work longer hours yet still have good productivity. Because of a balanced organ system, better flow of energy and blood from daily practice of taiji and qigong, the immune system is balanced. I have seen many students improve their energy levels and immune systems. They rarely catch colds. Even when they have caught colds, they recover quickly.

Effects on the Nervous System

As mentioned above, the movements from taiji and qigong affect the nervous system, including the central nervous system, peripheral nervous system, and autonomic nervous system. These whole-body exercises incorporate breathing and mental focus, which allows qi and blood to flow better to all parts of the body, including the brain. The biochemicals and neurochemicals in the body and brain therefore become balanced, and you can be more focused, learn more quickly, think more logically, maintain mental sharpness and alertness, and perform daily tasks with greater ease.

Taiji and qigong not only regulate the somatic nervous system (responsible for voluntary movement of the skeletal muscles), as evidenced by the improved mobility of the muscles and joints, but also improve the autonomic nervous system, including sympathetic and parasympathetic nervous system response. As we discussed previously, the autonomic nervous system is made up of the sympathetic and parasympathetic nervous systems and is divided into two opposite functions. These neural networks control the internal organ systems, glands, blood vessels, and sensory systems.

For many years, my focus has been on the nervous system and restoring autonomic nervous function. The healing work I do and the special exercises I create are designed to improve and balance the entire nervous system. As we know, the nervous system functions like a government of the whole body.

Each deep inhalation stimulates sympathetic activity, whereas each exhalation stimulates parasympathetic activity. The more regulated breathing you practice, the better-balanced autonomic nervous system you will have. That is why qigong masters have much fewer physical complaints. They have very good digestion, mental clarity, and immune function. This helps explains how taiji and qigong have a self-regulating effect on the human body.

There will be more details about the autonomic nervous system in a coming chapter, but I want to point out here that these benefits remain even as you age, which has given me the encouragement to write the book *Brain Fitness*. I have seen many of my friends with declining memories, even some who were very smart at a younger age. On the other hand, I have noticed that my taiji and qigong students have less depression and anxiety, less stress, and less confusion when making decisions. It greatly benefits people who have attention deficit disorder (ADD), too. I believe if we start to teach children taiji or qigong at early ages, it could help them to focus, and they would do better in their academic studies and other activities. They would have healthier mental processes too. Unfortunately, our culture has not paid much attention to this, so it is not generally supported.

Correction of Chemical Imbalances

Deep, slow, and regulated breathing along with body movement help to harmonize the body's chemistry, including adrenaline, noradrenaline, serotonin, and hormones. Many illnesses are caused by chemical or hormonal imbalances. We often use external chemicals to balance the internal chemicals, such as taking medication to supplement a chemical that is low in the blood. I disagree with this approach, and here is why: our body has an autoregulating system, which allows us to be in balance most of the time. If a certain chemical is low, the autoregulating system will stimulate the corresponding organs or glands to release more of this particular chemical to bring it to a normal level. But sometimes low levels can just be temporary and soon return to normal. Just like if we have a cold one day and feel better just a few days later. External chemicals (or pills) suppress this self-regulating response and provide false information to the body, so it stops releasing the chemical it needs. That is why a person who takes a thyroid hormone pill will usually have to take it for life. If a person uses a pill to supplement the thyroid hormone, the destruction of the self-regulating system of the thyroid gland, pituitary gland, and hypothalamus can occur. The result is that the thyroid no longer functions. If, on the other hand, the person starts to practice taiji, qigong, or other exercises consistently—or gets natural treatment such as with Chinese herbs—this person has a chance of restoring the self-regulating system. Eventually, the hormone level can return to normal.

Other Benefits

- Both taiji and qigong improve metabolism. You rarely see an overweight qigong master or longtime practitioner.

- Improved balance and coordination, which research has shown helps to prevent falls and injuries.

- Cancer healing—this is a result of taiji and qigong's ability to improve the functioning of the immune system and strengthen organ energy, both of which are crucial for fighting cancer. I know very few people believe this statement. A majority of people may say, "Yeah, right, Doc. This is a joke. Cancer needs chemotherapy, radiation therapy, hormone therapy, steroid therapy, surgery, and drugs." Sound familiar? But think about it for a moment: how many cancer patients died even though they had received these conventional therapies? Treating cancer has two components: killing the cancer cells and strengthening/nourishing the body. Conventional medicine only kills the cancer cells. But when you kill cancer cells, the body's own cells get damaged too. This is why we need qigong and taiji to strengthen and nourish the body, which helps it repair, heal, and balance its immune system. This is the second part of treating cancer. Many of us already know that most cancer patients lose their life from infection due to a weakened immune system, not from cancer itself. I will discuss qigong and cancer in greater detail in a future book.

In China, people who have cancer always seek treatment from both approaches to medicine: conventional and holistic. Most of them do qigong regularly in addition to using herbal medicine. I asked several cancer patients to practice qigong in addition to visiting me regularly; they had very good results—some are even cancer-free. I highly recommend that people who have cancer make qigong or taiji a lifelong practice. They will not regret it.

How Taiji and Qigong Prevent Brain Aging and Memory Loss

As we age, our bodies slow down, and we tend to become forgetful. The good news is that research has shown that regular physical exercise and other health-promoting practices can maintain and even restore our memory function and learning ability. I have been experimenting with this my whole life in an effort to support my health, learning, memory, and overall self-improvement. My goal is to avoid dementia and physical disability and to be able to enjoy my life for as long as I can. There is also clinical science to support what my hypothesis tells me is possible.

Qigong started four thousand years ago and taiji started four hundred years ago. Their popularity comes from their effectiveness in healing, prevention, and slowing down the aging process, especially brain aging. From thousands of years of experience, people in China know why they need to do certain things for their health and how to do them, and then they just do them. By "just doing it," they get results, and they learn from the results. If there are negative outcomes, they make corrections for next time. If there are positive results, they continue to improve. Not everything that works can be explained. In the West, people seem to require scientific answers to "why" and "how" questions before they take action. But things appear to be changing. More and more of the younger generations are willing to try things and learn from trying; in that way, they find out "why" and "how." This is what I call activating the brain from doing things. The more we do, the more we understand the "why" and the "how."

Using taiji and qigong to prevent brain aging is presented here from my own experience, including the changing behaviors and attitudes seen in my students, as well as the observations of many masters in China. I have summarized these below.

1. LIFELONG LEARNING

Learning should never stop. I always tell my family—and say the same thing in my lectures and other speaking engagements—"the day you stop learning is the day you stop living." Learning is a big part of healing; healing is a big part of learning. Taiji involves learning. When you start to learn things you didn't know, you begin to shift your focus to new knowledge, new approaches, new movements, and a new lifestyle. Taiji learning is continuous and multileveled in skill, depth, and meaning. Through continuous learning and practice, you will get the meaningful part—the true nature of taiji. If you are just starting as a beginner, you will feel good immediately from the practice of relaxation. If you are an advanced student, you will feel good continuously from the sustained practice of energy fluidity. Either way, you get benefits. Even people who do it incorrectly still get benefits. As you practice for more than a year or two, your taiji form will become more graceful and beautiful, and you will feel like you are dancing on the clouds. This gives you an added feeling of accomplishment and satisfaction. Learning taiji is challenging, but the challenge will help you enhance brain plasticity, which will support you as you age.

Any kind of challenge is stimulation for our brains. Without challenge, we would never be able to invent things. Without challenge, our lives would not advance. If we rely on a calculator all the time, soon we can't calculate easy equations anymore. If we store every phone number in our cell phone contacts list or computer, we won't be able to dial those numbers ourselves. In one scientific study on aging and the brain, scientists confirmed that *any* intellectually challenging activity and *any* activity involving mildly complex movement stimulate the growth of dendrites, and this adds more connections in the brain's neural pathways.

When you work on learning taiji or qigong, you are shifting gears to a higher level of positive energy. The more positive energy you have, the more improvement you will see in all aspects of your life and being. The positive energy also goes to your brain, and therefore all of your body parts function better.

Just as there are two halves to the brain, there are two types of thought: conscious and unconscious. Conscious thought involves your awareness of your surroundings, your agenda for the day, plans for work or travel, your pleasures, and your peeves. You can logically rearrange, discuss, and guide your behavior according to your needs. Unconscious thoughts, on the other hand, are more spontaneously occurring and out of your intentional control, such as holding a cup, saying good night to your spouse, and your heart beating fast when you are nervous. Taiji practice raises the quality of your conscious thought processes, empowering you to be more in tune with your daily experiences.

2. A BREAK IN YOUR ROUTINE

We grow up with certain fixed routines and most of us don't want to change those routines. Such routines can not only include our diet, how we do our jobs, and the way we interact with people but also habitual ways of thinking. We don't like to do something if we are not familiar with it. While on a hiking trip with my sister and my husband in Acadia National Park, we got disoriented in the woods. My sister and I wanted to explore for a way out, but my husband insisted that we go back the same way to get out. Seeing his anxiety, I almost gave up and agreed to go back the same way. Suddenly, my sister found a new path. It guided us onto another main path, and we found our way back. She broke the routine and helped us find a new path out of the woods. We drive on the same road every day because the familiarity of the road is comforting. But if we never try a different road, we'll never find a better route. Sometimes new roads are shortcuts or help us avoid traffic jams.

Routines can be brain deadening. When something unusual happens that gets us out of our routine, we get anxious; we don't know what to do. We feel like our brains are not working. Just think, many of us go to work every day, come home, eat, sleep, go to work the next day—our brains are programmed in such a way that we don't even have to think anymore. Our brain cells don't get stimulated and certain neural pathways shut down. *Breaking the routine is a brain fitness workout.* This allows new activities for the brain to be activated and encourages brain cells to communicate, opening new neural pathways. Watching TV is another brain-killing activity; however, this doesn't mean we need to give up on TV. I like to watch the news, some nature programs, and other educational programs. But research has shown that when we watch TV, the brain is less active, even less active than during sleep. When you are watching TV, your brain is passive—or active in a passive way. Some TV programs can even traumatize the brain, which can make us unable to view things as a whole. If you know how to balance your life, you will be careful to watch TV wisely and add other brain fitness exercises into your life. Think for a moment: how many smart "couch potatoes" are there? (Although I don't mean to say that all people who watch TV are couch potatoes.)

Taiji exercise and learning are not familiar to most Americans. We did not grow up with slow-motion exercises. We like fast and vigorous. We like *pain*. We often hear, "No pain, no gain." This is not an entirely accurate statement. Not all that long ago, human beings may have had to struggle just to survive. But things are different now;

we don't have to suffer too much to get what we need. There has been so much change in our lives, our health, our society, our government, our technology, our earth, our lifestyle, our science, and more. That old statement about pain and gain also needs to change. Our needs go beyond surviving and just making a living. Physical burdens have been replaced with mental ones. We need tools to help us to relieve the mental burdens. In other words, even exercise in this modern lifestyle should be balanced—fast *and* slow movements. The yin energy (receptive, slow) and the yang energy (active, fast) should be evident everywhere to keep our lives balanced. Many of our problems are caused by the imbalance of yin and yang. However, it is true that hard work, smart learning, and dedication can lead you to success.

Once you open your mind, you can purposely derail your routine and adjust your old habits. You can build brain cells by choosing to experience a totally new concept, a new philosophy, a new way of life, a new journey. Your brain cells will have to branch out to make new connections with other brain cells.

I keep saying that taiji is a journey. That's because you are always learning new things from taiji practice, acquiring new knowledge, experiencing new feelings, making new movements or understanding old movements more deeply, forging new friendships, and building new energy. Taiji opens your mind and shows you a pathway to a new way of seeing things.

3. BETTER, DEEPER SLEEP

We know sleeping disorders can accelerate aging, especially brain aging. The first thing you notice about people with sleep problems is that they look tired. The next thing you notice is that their speech is slow. This indicates that the brain language center is sluggish and less active. The same is true for other parts of the brain. We have all had the experience that if we don't sleep well the previous night, our minds are not clear, our memory is not sharp, and we cannot concentrate. The sleep-deprived brain has less ability to store new information and retrieve old information. I struggled with a sleeping disorder in medical school. This couldn't have helped my memory problems. The day I graduated, I said to myself, *I never want to go back to school again*, even though I hadn't done poorly at all.

Many of my patients with sleeping problems tell me, "My brain is in a fog" or "I can't remember things." If a person has had a long-term sleeping disorder, you can see that she looks older than she actually is. A good night's sleep is also an important part of healing from many illnesses. Just think about a machine: if used nonstop, the machine soon breaks down.

With regular practice of taiji and qigong, your neurochemicals are brought into balance and your body's electricity and sleep become regulated. Your brain is no longer exhausted and you are more alert. Now brain healing can begin.

4. INCREASED OXYGEN

I often mention oxygen in my lectures, speeches, classes, trainings, and conversations. This is because it is so important to life and health. Our brain, although only about 2 percent of our body weight, consumes roughly 20 percent of the oxygen we breathe. When the brain is nurtured with adequate oxygen, it helps to bring better function to the breathing center, vascular center, and all other centers. If you have problems with your heart and lungs that affect your breathing and oxygen level, it will also affect your brain's oxygen level. Cognitive power declines when there is a decreased supply of oxygen to the brain. This is why you see an older person get cranky no matter how much you try to make things clear. This may also sometimes show in a senior's stubbornness.

When I see a person yawn too many times, I tease him, saying, "You need more oxygen." When I see a person who sleeps too much, I say it quietly: "You need more oxygen." When I see a person driving and feeling sleepy, I may also say, "You need more oxygen." When I see a person feeling tired all the time: "You need more oxygen." This is because I know that low oxygen levels can affect a person in many ways.

As we know, the brain must consume oxygen to be able to function. It is the lungs that help us get oxygen through the breath. If your brain lacks oxygen for six to nine minutes, your brain can be damaged. If you lack oxygen for twenty minutes, you will die. If your body lacks food for fifteen days, you may still live. The oxygen to our brain is very important. If your brain has enough oxygen, you are most likely alert; if your brain lacks oxygen, you feel tired, lethargic, and overwhelmed by the mental fog. You will also notice that when you are tired or feel sleepy, you feel a little clearer after a big yawn. Yawning is the deepest breath we can take; we do it to get oxygen to our tired brains.

We now understand that one of the most important parts of preventing brain aging is getting enough oxygen to it. Practicing qigong and taiji involves deep breathing, which helps to bring more oxygen to your body and your brain; you will notice the change in the way you feel overall. You will feel less cloudy, fresher, more alert, and more energetic.

5. UNIQUE TAIJI MOVEMENT SEQUENCES

Taiji movements are not like any other exercise. The special choreographed movements are circular and in constant motion. Many gestures cross the body from left to right, from upward to downward, and from right diagonal to left diagonal. It is multi-dimensional. The footwork is slow, on the diagonal, well controlled, and involves multiple changing stances. Through these changing stances and whole-body movements, multidimensional both spatially and the internally, you learn to be more aware of your body. You become aware of your tension, your balance, your energy, your emotional stability, and your visual surroundings. You pay attention to your energy center and are able to self-correct your posture. You know if you are off-center or if you lose your balance. You move with your intention, and you move your body while your mind experiences calm and peace.

Taiji movement stimulates the senses, the faculty of motor control, the sense of spatial orientation, the sense of balance and equilibrium, the forebrain and hindbrain, and the left and right brain. It also provides cross-brain stimulation. The whole brain is stimulated. Taiji movements are very good brain fitness exercises. We use aerobic exercise to increase our heart rate and promote better circulation. We also need brain fitness exercises to improve our brain function and learning abilities. Western science has confirmed that movement is crucial to brain health and definitely affects cognitive change. Eastern practitioners knew it all along.

Evidence shows that movement is also crucial to every other brain function, including memory, emotion, language, learning, and more. Try to do qigong for three to five minutes when you are tired after working, or writing a paper if you are a student, and your brain can't seem to think anymore. You will be able to return to work refreshed or put more words on paper. What is happening here? Our higher brain functions evolved from lower functions involving basic mobility, and these higher functions still depend on the lower ones. A sedentary lifestyle promotes brain aging—too much TV or any other "brain dead" couch-potato activity.

The well-known kinesiology and learning researcher Dr. Paul Dennison, along with his wife, movement educator Gail Dennison, have developed a movement program that has been proven to exercise the brain. They call it Brain Gym. Brain Gym is a movement-based technique to enhance learning ability for children who have learning difficulties in conventional settings. As we age, we do not learn as quickly or as well as younger people. The information takes longer to put into memory storage, and it takes longer to learn new things. Studies have shown that we shift from being visual and auditory learners to *kinesthetic* learners. That is, we don't absorb so much from reading or listening as we once did; we need to learn by doing. Above and beyond this learning style, Brain Gym has helped to establish even stronger links between certain kinds of movement techniques and enhancing brain function in general. The exercise movements from taiji and qigong can help adults achieve maximum learning and delay the brain-aging process.

I have a friend named Nancy. Nancy's husband has several electronics systems hooked into the television and therefore needs several different remotes. In order to watch TV, she has to use several buttons on each remote. Even though her husband has taught her several times, she still cannot find the right button to turn on the TV. Finally, she just bought another TV with only one remote. Many older people have trouble using multisystem entertainment centers. Here is an opposite story. One of my taiji students studied piano at the age of fifty-eight. She told me that her piano teacher was amazed at her ability to learn. My own experience was learning cello; I didn't start until I was forty-nine. I was skeptical myself! But now I realize I can learn, and I even improve. It makes me feel good to see that improvement.

With certain body movements to stimulate neural pathways, you enable nerve cells to communicate with one another and create more activity in the brain network. The participant feels more alert and can easily put memory into storage and later retrieve the information. That is why we say taiji enhances learning ability.

Taiji and qigong movements balance both sides of the brain by encouraging cross-connections with information between the left and right brain. With this special training, our dominant side can become more cooperative with the other, fostering a greater balance between the two sides. This hemispheric balance helps you to develop well-balanced cognitive, communication, and social skills. Once your brain is more balanced, you may even be more pleasant with your partner or companion, more easygoing, better able to multitask, more even-tempered, have an increased ability to learn new things, and be less rigid or stubborn. These are some of the changes I have observed firsthand in many of my students.

The cross-brain movements create a sort of cross-brain training. The stimulation causes more communication to occur through synapses of the brain cells. This enhanced connection and communication between the brain cells keeps our brains young and our memory strong.

Science has also confirmed that taiji improves the body's balance. The cerebellum controls balance, coordination, adjustment, and smoothing out of movement. Taiji improves the cerebellum's function, bringing about better coordination and balance.

Recent studies have shown that the cerebellum is not just related to movement but also to cognition. For those with injuries to the brain and cerebellum, there are studies that suggest a possibility for healing from taiji and qigong practice. Because taiji improves cerebellum function, it is likely practice of the art will improve both physical balance and cognitive skill. By rewiring the brain itself, not only can the brain learn new tricks, but it can also change its structure and function, even in old age. Taiji is truly a brain fitness regimen for adults.

6. BALANCE AND THE AUTONOMIC NERVE SYSTEM

I mentioned before that the human body is controlled by the nervous system, and all *organs* are controlled by the autonomic nervous system. Many illnesses are caused by disorders of these systems.

Autonomic nerve impulses originate in the central nervous system and perform the most basic human functions automatically, without conscious control. Autonomic nerve fibers exiting from the central nervous system form the sympathetic, the parasympathetic, and the enteric nervous systems. The actions of the sympathetic and parasympathetic systems often oppose each other. For example, sympathetic nerves are responsible for increasing the heart rate, raising blood pressure, and causing us to breathe harder. The parasympathetic nerves do the opposite: decrease heart rate, reduce blood pressure, and slow down breath. The sympathetic system is involved in "fight and flight" responses while the parasympathetic division is involved in "rest and digest" actions that do not require an immediate response.

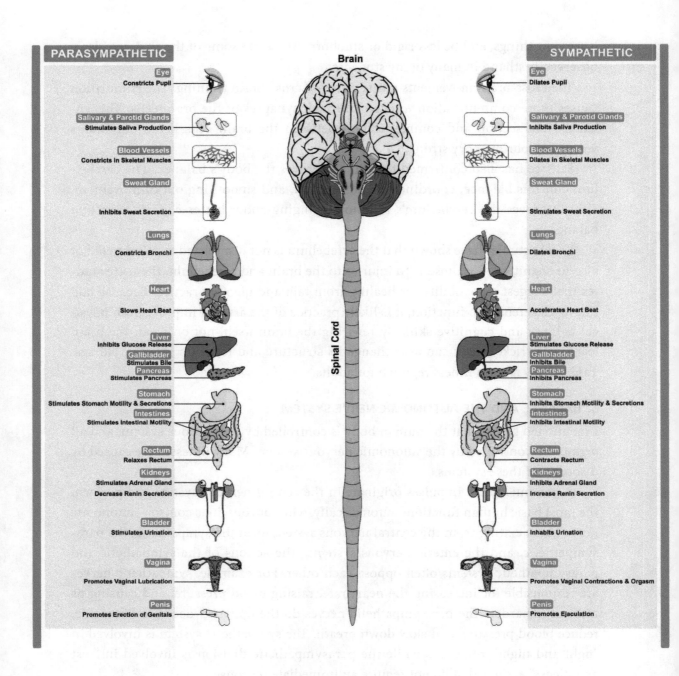

The sympathetic nervous system connects the internal organs to the brain. It responds to stress by increasing heart rate and blood flow to the muscles and decreasing blood flow to the skin. The parasympathetic nervous system increases digestive secretions and slows the heartbeat. Both systems give feedback to the central nervous system about the condition of internal organs to help maintain the body's equilibrium.

The autonomic nervous system controls the irises and the muscles involved in the functioning of the heart, lungs, stomach, and other organs. It is in charge of the automatic functions—those we have no control over. These include the beating of the heart, digestion, breathing, and sexual arousal. Emotions strongly influence the autonomic system. For example, anger makes your heart beat faster, and anxiety can interfere with digestion.

Patients visit their doctors for unexplained symptoms, and they are disappointed when doctors cannot find anything wrong and cannot help them. These unexplained ailments are most likely caused by disorders of the autonomic nervous system. When I correct the imbalance of an autonomic disorder, patients' symptoms diminish and patients feel better. When they call me a "miracle worker," I just tell them what I did: regulated autonomic function. The autonomic nervous system has a close relation to the meridian system in Chinese medicine. I love working with the nervous systems, especially the autonomic nervous system because people can feel the difference right away.

The movements in taiji and qigong, along with warm-up exercises involving twisting and turning of the body, loosen the spine and all of the vertebra joints. This makes the paired peripheral nerves of the spine work in harmony, balancing the autonomic nervous system and therefore maintaining homeostasis in the body and brain. Deep and slow breathing stimulate the respiratory and circulatory centers in the brain, helping to regulate autonomic function.

7. BUILDING STRONG QI, STRENGTHENING ALL ORGANS

Qi is vital energy, or life force. It is the energy that underlies everything in the universe. Qi in the human body refers to the various types of bioenergy associated with human health and vitality. Changing qi in our body can affect our health and well-being. Qi is present internally and externally and controls the function of all parts of the body. There are many different types of qi in the body. These are discussed in my first book, *Natural Healing with Qigong* (YMAA, 2004).

Taiji and qigong build stronger qi in the body and promote qi flow in the body. The strong and smooth flow of qi helps to strengthen all of the organs—kidneys, heart, liver, spleen, and lungs. In traditional Chinese medicine, the word *kidney* is related to the brain, bone, and bone marrow. As noted above, it also stores jing (essence, also called fundamental substance). The word *heart* is related to shen (spirit), mind, and also the brain. The word *liver* is related to emotions and moods and has an association with the brain as well. The spleen is associated with digestion, absorption, metabolism, and blood—all of which bring nutrients to the brain. The lung governs the breath and brings more oxygen to the brain. As you can see, all of the organs are associated with the brain. Because the body and the brain are connected, by exercising the brain, you help the body. By exercising the body, you help the brain.

Working with qi in the body is like working with an electric power plant. We use the electricity generated by the power plant to enable us to create, produce, and perform all kinds of things. By elevating body energy with taiji or qigong, we can stimulate the brain and body to create, produce, and perform all kinds of things as well. Qi is fundamental to everything. For centuries, Eastern philosophers have known the connection between our minds and our bodies—this is the basis of qigong. All three components of qi practice—mental focus, body movement, and breath—affect our brain. The mind focuses to help us memorize. With a scattered mind, you lose memory. Body movements, together with deep breathing, help the energy flow through the body smoothly, finally reaching and passing through the brain, a finely tuned, biological supercomputer. At this point, our body's energy system reaches equilibrium.

With a taiji workout, your energy pathways are opened, your internal organs start to work harmoniously, and your mind and body begin to work together. You are more adept, more open to learning, more willing to try and to experience. Your brain cells start to communicate. Each new thing you do makes more connections among brain cells. This harmonious energy also promotes rapid healing of illness.

8. BALANCING THE EMOTIONS

The right and the left frontal lobes are very important for the regulation of emotion. They are needed for making decisions in both the social and personal realms. Because taiji stimulates the whole brain, it coordinates the left and right brain and stimulates the crisscrossing of information between the left and the right brains and the upper and lower brains. It also balances the limbic system, also known as the emotion center. Neurotransmitters start flowing smoothly between the synapses.

Taiji balances emotion also by developing self-awareness, focus, positive thinking, and building strong qi. Emotional balance is very important to prevent brain aging and provides a good physical and mental environment for learning. Having balanced emotions enables you to be focused and pay attention to what you are doing. This helps both learning and memory. An impaired emotional state can reduce learning ability and make a person prone to memory loss.

Many people use medication to treat emotional problems; I disagree with this approach. People want an easy solution and a shortcut for their health issues. They don't realize that certain medications can cause memory loss, brain fog, brain aging, and sometimes even sudden death.

A friend of mine, a very sweet and smart person, is dealing with an emotional issue. She has been suffering from depression for a long time and is on medications. One of the issues I have noticed with her is that she has a hard time remembering things, especially appointments and dates. This became a problem for me as well when I made special arrangements to meet with her, and she forgot that she was supposed to see me.

9. INVOLVEMENT IN MARTIAL ARTS

We all know that martial arts practice is intended to make you strong and disciplined. Martial arts can give you mental power that helps you achieve. In almost every form of taiji, there is some martial arts relevance. People choose to practice taiji for different reasons: to find inner peace, for stress relief, for flexibility, for healing, for longevity, for increasing energy and stamina, or for competition and self-defense. Taiji originated as a martial art, and some movements are more pronounced in their martial aspect and can be used for self-defense. These martial arts movements make you feel stronger, more powerful, and more in control of yourself. They give you a solid, safe, stable, and determined feeling. They make you feel good and help you believe in yourself, which helps you succeed in anything you want to do. Whatever you do, you need to feel good about yourself. You cannot succeed if you don't feel good about yourself.

10. CHOOSING THE RIGHT MUSIC

Music is everywhere. We listen to music when we drive, walk, work out in the gym, sit in the doctor's or natural therapist's waiting room, or just relax at home. Music is important in our lives. Different music has different effect on people. Certain music can have healing effects, while some loud, noisy music can have negative effects on our heart, mind, and blood pressure. Some music can even make you more depressed, sad, and anxious. Younger people like fast and stimulating music, while older people and those with heart disease like slow and relaxing music. Rock and roll won't work for taiji practice. Science has fully demonstrated the effects of music on our brains and on our health. Many studies have even shown that certain music can reduce tension and enhance specific types of intelligence, such as verbal ability and spatial-temporal reasoning.

In general, the music used in taiji practice is relaxing, gentle, calming, and tranquil. Adding music to taiji and qigong practice gives double benefits for well-being. Using relaxing music helps you slow the movements down and become more aware of your movement, relaxation, and feeling of unity. If you try to use different music, the results of practice may be different.

11. RESPONDING TO RELAXATION

I have treated numerous patients who were loaded with stress. I cannot say that I don't have any stress, but I can say that taiji and qigong help me to manage it well most of the time. In addition, they help me remain focused on what I am doing. If we carry a lot of stress, there is less blood flowing to our muscles and our brain. Our muscles become weakened, we feel tired, and our brain is fatigued. This can be proven with muscle-testing techniques (such as a kinesiology test). I cannot write when I am stressed because I cannot focus and form a complete sentence. When I look at my writing after, I say to myself, "This does not make any sense." You may recall a time when you were stressed and could not think straight. When you carry stress for a long time, eventually your muscles will degenerate, and you will feel pain all over your body. Your doctor then might give you a diagnosis called fibromyalgia. You may think that's the answer, but it's not. You only have a name, a word that does not mean anything. The real answer is yourself, your participation in healing. If I were to give your condition a name, it would be poor circulation, chronic inflammation, and degeneration in the muscle tissue. I have treated many people with "fibromyalgia" who took many different kinds of medications or painkillers but still had the pain after the painkillers wore off. Many of these people develop other problems from the side effects of their medications. We now understand that to help fibromyalgia, the first thing is to get your blood and energy moving.

There are many ailments related to stress or tension over long periods, such as insomnia, headache, heart disease, hypertension, cholesterol, gastrointestinal problems, sexual dysfunction, back problems, neck problems, inability to focus, and more. In addition, stress causes distractions. You lose focus, and you lose your normal sense of what life is supposed to be like.

There are two things that can truly manage stress: wisdom and the practice of it. Wisdom helps you understand the stress and find the right solution to best deal with it without harming the mind or body. Putting your wisdom into practice means working toward the ability to relieve stress instantaneously.

When you practice taiji and qigong, you are practicing "meditation in motion," the best relaxation exercise for relief of stress. This also helps to relieve symptoms of anxiety, panic, heart palpitation, and high blood pressure. When you feel relaxed, you get the sensation that all the stress is melting away. Your body has less tension. You feel calmer and more peaceful. The relaxation you get from taiji or qigong practice allows your energy to move smoothly through the body—your overwhelmed brain gets a rest, your muscles relax, your emotions settle down, and your tiredness disappears. You feel balanced. Once your muscles are relaxed, more blood flows into the muscle tissue, helping your muscles to grow stronger. You become more comfortable, more aware of yourself in time and space. You become more conscious of where you hold the tension or feel the weakness, and eventually, you try to find ways to heal yourself. Now you've got something tangible to work on, which then restores your sense of what life is supposed to be like. Once you are more relaxed, you are more positive. Your positive state of mind helps you heal your chronic or old wound.

12. BECOMING ROOTED

With our modern lifestyle, we are distracted by so many activities and overwhelming information. We don't know how to focus or how to find what we are really attracted to. If you ask college students, even older ones, what they really want, many of them won't know how to answer. Some of them might just go for whatever job they can find to make a living, and others go for a high-paying job. But what if it turns out that they are not happy with the money-making job?

Taiji and qigong help you feel rooted, stable, and focused, allowing you to find your passion. This kind of practice helps you become more aware of yourself and your spirit. It makes you more able to listen to your heart and soul. Taiji brings you closer to nature; it helps you think and act more naturally, more authentically. The more natural you are, the more you understand universal energy and how it works. Doing things in a natural way is part of the brain's learning pattern, and getting away from technology sometimes can be a great benefit or relief. We eventually find what we truly want, what we are attracted to, what we do best, and what makes us happy. When you do a job you feel good about, the feeling is priceless. There is a saying: "Less is more." Being in tune with nature, you cannot go wrong. Being rooted brings great advantages.

13. TOUCHING

Touching can be very therapeutic. Sometimes we rub sore muscles when we feel discomfort. Sometimes we massage our temple areas when we get headaches. If we fall and hurt a foot or leg, we use our hands to press on the injured area. If your child has a headache, the first thing you do is touch his head to feel if he has a fever. You then rub his head, trying to make him feel better. Why is that? It is because touching eases dis-ease. Touching can bring special benefits to our body, mind, and brain. Neuroscientists can see the effect of touching on the brain using functional magnetic resonance imaging (fMRI). There is an increase in blood flow that is correlated with an increase in neuronal activity. Touch appears to affect multiple brain regions at conscious and unconscious levels. Touch has a wide range of impacts on the brain, influencing our sensations, movements, thought processes, and capacity to learn new movements.

Some of the warm-up exercises and qigong forms involve self-massage and acupressure. Through these kinds of sensory stimulations, along with body movement, mental focus, and deep breathing, not only do our brains get immediate benefit, but our total awareness is also heightened. Our bodies' acupressure points are the stations of the energy pathway. You are delivering qi to these stations when you perform self-massage in qigong practice.

14. GROUP ENERGY

As we discussed above, one of the highlights of taiji and qigong is that creates a nice social gathering; we call it a qi gathering. Human beings have always enjoyed participating in group activities, group functions, group performances, and other social events. Human beings are social beings. There are thousands of associations, professional societies, churches, and study groups. People seek others like themselves to do the things they enjoy, to enrich their lives and spirits. Social activity brings a learning experience with it; the more you interact with people, the more you learn. Animals are the same—like a wolf that is part of a pack. Scientists are finding that animals raised in an enriched environment have at least twice as many new brain cells in the region of the brain responsible for memory and learning as the control group. The stimulation of their environment also provoked the development of new connections (synapses) between neurons. In addition, they found that animals that live in an enriched environment live longer.

Taiji draws together like-minded people just as other groups do. If you like to chat, you gravitate toward chatty people. If you are religious, you seek out a religious group or participate in church functions. If you enjoy the outdoors, you find other outdoorsy people and do outdoor activities with them. If you enjoy being healthy and living a stress-free lifestyle, you can find taiji and qigong groups. As long as you know what you are looking for in a group, you can find one that suits your interests. The best part about taiji and qigong groups is that they are easygoing, flexible, adaptable, kind, tolerant, and smart. They learn taiji and qigong, and they follow Daoist practice by focusing on health, happiness, and longevity.

Scientific research has repeatedly proven that social deprivation has severe negative effects on overall cognitive ability. Not only that, social deprivation can cause depression, anxiety, and other serious illnesses. Many people exercise daily by themselves. They use the treadmill or elliptical machine, lift weights, walk, or run. They don't have to interact with anyone else. In the gym, each person usually works on individual muscle groups, one at a time. Many people want to increase their heart rate using treadmills or work up a sweat to increase metabolism in hopes of losing weight. Everyone has a different purpose for going to the gym. There is nothing wrong with these activities; they are better than doing nothing. Any kind of exercise is beneficial. However, with taiji and qigong, it is different. Group energy is important, and you get two for the price of one—exercise and socializing. Whether practiced in a classroom or outdoors, taiji develops a great deal of group energy. Group practice fosters discussion, friendship, social connection, group harmony, and all of the positive traits you get from the group. Beyond just having fun, the combination of taiji and group energy makes you feel great. It is no wonder it is so helpful in preventing memory loss and enhancing learning ability. For many years I had observed that our students who came to taiji class felt happy, joyful, comfortable, and relaxed. This was when I had my taiji school (New England School of Tai Chi) in Massachusetts. Currently in Florida, my focus is on training taiji instructors in a group setting. Yet the same phenomenon occurs after the teachers complete my full training course together.

Students tend to do better when they practice together because the energy of each individual affects the energy of others in the class. When everyone's energy channels are open, the whole classroom is loaded with energy. You cannot see this, but you can feel it. In any kind of work, teamwork always brings the best results. The harmonious group energy makes you feel good for a long time.

This is what one of my students said:

As a young man, I could run a marathon and ride my bicycle for one hundred miles. After I ran the Boston Marathon, I felt I had made my way to the top of the mountain: I did something that most people will never be able to physically do, for whatever reasons those may be. Even though I was in good physical shape, after starting my journey with taiji, I realized I had trouble coordinating my body in certain ways.

Since then and with much dedicated practice, I have improved my coordination tremendously. And I have humbly realized I am not at the top of the mountain but only at the beginning of a path!

Taiji has not only helped me physically but mentally and spiritually as well. I have been stuck in a dead-end retail environment for the past six years. Through the influence of taiji and qigong classes, I am now going to school to be a holistic health counselor. . . . I believe my journey in taiji so far has empowered me to utilize a part of myself that was just lying dormant.

Therefore, even as a young man, I can personally attest to the all-encompassing well-being benefits of this awesome exercise!

—Mark G.

In China it is easy to practice outdoors because there are so many people exercising in public parks or other public places. It automatically draws you into the group, and you blend into the practice. It is harder to do taiji by yourself outdoors in America. Not only because it is such a new and different exercise here, but also because people feel self-conscious doing this kind of exercise in a public place. Normally, we only see activities like walking, jogging, biking, or playing sports done outside. But I recommend you try to do qigong or taiji outdoors. You may be surprised to find out how good you feel.

Please keep in mind that taiji and qigong are not magic, even though they can provide amazing, miraculous benefits. All the benefits come from diligent learning, practice, belief, a positive attitude, and patience. It is a lifestyle, a journey, and a way.

CHAPTER 3

The Difference between Taiji and Qigong

WHAT IS THE DIFFERENCE between taiji and qigong?" This is a question people ask all the time. In the United States, more people know taiji than qigong. They don't associate the two. They see them as separate Chinese practices. Also, more studies focus on taiji than qigong. The truth is that both taiji and qigong are internal energy workouts, but qigong is easier. They share the same principles and philosophies, and they offer similar health benefits. However, they do have their differences. Taiji has a four-hundred-year-old history; qigong's history stretches back more than four thousand years. As you can see, qigong is the grandfather of taiji.

Taiji is a type of qigong, a higher level of qigong that requires many years to learn to perform correctly. Like qigong, taiji requires concentration, but it also involves more coordination and motor skills. Generally speaking, taiji is much more challenging. It is a deeper qi practice and more fun than qigong, especially when you become more familiar with it. There are five main styles of taiji: Yang, Chen, Wu', Wu, and Sun. They look similar but differ in some details with different movements and different ways to enhance your qi. Chen style is the oldest, and Yang style is the easiest. The most popular style in China and the United States is the Yang style, followed by the Wu style, and the Chen style. The most powerful and closest related to gongfu is the Chen style. It is challenging to learn, and you need diligent practice. But once you understand the principles, you can apply them to martial arts and self-defense. All forms of taiji involve a qi practice or qi workout. That is why we call it a higher level of qigong.

Qigong is easier than taiji, and it also has many different forms. But some of them can be difficult. Some people think qigong is too boring and not challenging enough. This is because they don't really know qigong well and haven't practiced it properly. Either they may not have a good teacher, or they may have ADD and cannot pay attention. Qigong is not boring at all. If you practice qigong correctly, it is not easy. It

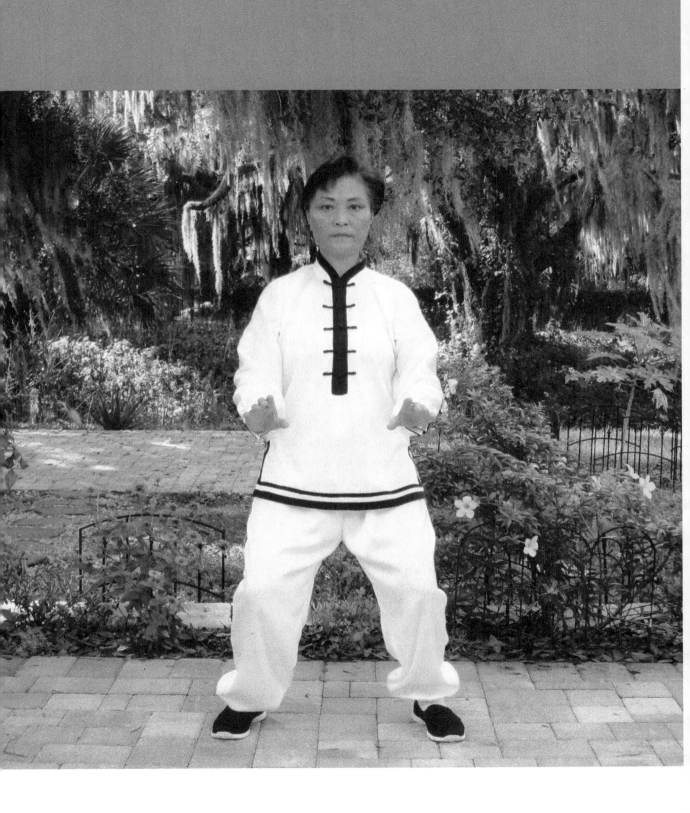

requires focus and control. However, certain types of qigong are easier than others. Some qigong forms are purely sitting in meditation and working on your mind and breath. Some forms work on your body while others work on breath and mind in addition to the body.

You should not separate these two exercises. Rather, think of them as brother and sister. In my class, I sometimes use qigong as a warm-up before taiji practice, and most students love it. I sometimes use taiji movements in qigong practice and have my students feel the qi as energy in their body and hands. People who practice taiji will sense the qi sooner when they practice qigong. People who practice qigong will learn taiji more quickly and more easily. Both come from the same family and are rooted in the Daoist practice of going with the flow.

If you are a beginner, I suggest you practice qigong first and, after you feel its benefits, then start to learn taiji. This way, you will know that qi does exist and can be felt. But there are no restrictions; do as you wish. If you start with taiji first, please do not be frustrated. You should feel no frustration when learning taiji. Remember this philosophy: go with the flow, and you'll be doing it right. Taiji is not about mechanical performance of movements but rather about undertaking a journey—a long journey maybe, but an amazing one that you won't regret.

Both taiji and qigong can be used to heal the body and mind, to nurture the spirit, to strengthen internal energy, to boost the immune system, and to help you focus. Both of them can be your lifetime friends. But there are some differences between taiji and qigong, which I will list here for reference.

PLEASE NOTE

The above comes from my own experience, but things are not black and white. The interpretation is not intended to be rigid, however; it is meant to be open-minded. You should experience both for yourself in order to really understand the benefits of each. You may discover something different and more valuable in one or the other. Everything has multiple aspects. Some things are good for one person, and other things are good for another person. Some exercises may be attractive to one person but may not be attractive to other people. My recommendation is that you try them for yourself and feel the differences. Don't be afraid of trying.

Taiji	Qigong
Advanced level of internal energy practice.	Beginner level of internal energy practice.
Needs total relaxation.	Some qigong may alternate between relaxation and muscle tension.
Movements are slow and circular; may initially be difficult to learn. Takes longer time to learn.	Movements are simpler, easy to follow, easy to learn, repetitive. Some qigong involves self-massage.
Five main styles or forms, some variations.	Various forms, for different purposes.
Breathing is slow and deep with each movement. Some fa jin movement (in Chen style) requires fast breath out.	Breathing can be slow or fast. It varies among different forms.
Comes from martial arts; can be used for self-defense. For prevention, relaxation, total self-control, and empowerment.	Created for natural healing and prevention. For relaxation and assisting healing. Sometimes immediate results can be seen.
Practiced while standing.	Practiced in any position.
Not practical for severe illnesses.	Good even for those with severe illnesses and for all abilities, skill levels, and ages—no restrictions.
Easy for beginners to get frustrated because of difficult movements.	May be too simple for some people. Some may become bored, especially those with ADD or attention deficit hyperactivity disorder (ADHD).
Creates feelings of euphoria, calm, relaxation, being energized. But may see healing results more slowly because the movements are more difficult to perfect.	Creates feelings of euphoria, calm, relaxation, being energized. See results more quickly, such as less pain, better breathing, mental clarity.
A spiritual discipline. Also helps to develop self-discipline.	A self-healing practice in addition to a spiritual discipline.
Participants can be younger, but is for all.	Participants can be older or middle aged, but is for all.
Taiji is a higher level of qigong practice.	Qigong can be a beginner level of taiji.

Fundamental Principles of Taiji Practice

For good study and practice, you need to understand taiji's principles. Once you understand the principles, learning becomes easier. Your taiji journey will be smoother, and you will develop better skills through practice. Many people practice taiji, but few practice following the principles. Those who do take time to practice regularly. What I call "regularly" is practicing daily between forty-five minutes to an hour and a half. Only regular practice allows you to understand the principles of taiji at a deep level. Your body will be permeated with a sense of well-being, and your whole practice will become more powerful. People who do a good job of following the principles get more health benefits and experience better qi circulation. They develop better martial skill too. Most people practice taiji because they heard good things about it from the media, in an article, or in books. They want to give it a try. Many give up, though, because of the difficulty of the movements. The media do not provide details on how to practice correctly, and some taiji teachers may teach only the movements, not the principles. Lack of well-trained teachers can be another reason for people to quit practicing or drop the class.

Most masters take only dedicated students. The dedicated students are not many, especially in modern life when everyone is so busy. But still, there are some people who practice and are in tune with nature and natural energy—as you will be after reading and applying the material in this book.

Taiji is fun and enjoyable if practiced correctly, especially when it comes to push hands practice. Those who have followed the taiji principles are more difficult to push over. Push hands is more for younger people, generally under fifty years of age. But anyone at any age can practice push hands if they and their partners know how to do it the harmonious way, which makes it very pleasurable.

The taiji principles are treasures given to us by the masters over the centuries. They allow us to achieve proper taiji practice, reach higher levels of martial arts skill, build character, and receive many other benefits.

Taiji Mental State and Physical Postures

When you start a taiji practice, the first thing you need to be aware of is your posture from head to toe. Generally speaking, every part of you should be relaxed.

1. YOUR MIND

Your mind should be a peaceful oasis. Every time new students come to my class, I would ask them to focus only on relaxation, nothing else. Taiji is complicated enough—students cannot learn if they are tense, otherwise they tend to forget the movements. The body is tense because the mind is tense. That is why relaxation starts with the mind.

Mind clear: There is nothing in your mind except to be with the flow of taiji.

Mind focused: You are focused on your energy center, your shifting weight, and complete relaxation from head to toe. You know there is positive energy surrounding you, and you should not worry about anything. Your intention is to start to use taiji to generate energy and let that energy work for you and nurture you. If you are self-conscious and carry stress, you won't have an efficient practice. You can never practice taiji well if you focus on your problems or other distractions.

Taiji actually helps people with attention deficit problems; partly, the art develops concentration. Once your mind is relaxed, you can generate the intention of moving energy. Then, once you are breathing correctly, the movements come more naturally. But for beginners, the breath work is not emphasized due to the complexity of taiji movements. I have observed that most beginning students have a hard time relaxing. They are self-conscious about other people watching them, especially if they think they have poor coordination or learn slowly. In taiji practice, being self-conscious is a total waste of energy. Your classmates are not focusing on you; they are focusing only on themselves and their own energy. The teacher only wants you to relax. Good teachers will not overcorrect new students because nit-picking can be annoying and frustrating to beginners.

2. YOUR HEAD, EYES, AND MOUTH

Your head should be upright and naturally lifted, with your neck relaxed. With this posture, you will feel the lifted spirit and energy. You can imagine a string attached to the top of your head, right in the center, lifting your head up. If you are hunched, your body is floppy, your energy feels low, and your spirit is hard to sense.

Your eyes should be aware and generate mental intention. You should not look at the floor (which many beginner students do). Your eyes correspond with the arm or leg movement during practice, but do not stare at your hand or arm. Your eyes should be focused in the direction of your yang movement—the dominant part of your body in taiji movements. For example, suppose you punch with your right fist while your left fist is simply held by your side, without moving. Your right punch is a yang movement, while holding your left fist passively by your side is a yin "movement." You express the intent of the movement with your eye. Then you will feel that your taiji performance is alive with power. Your spirit is lifted, your qi is moving. Accomplished Chinese martial arts practitioners have a very good "spirit of the eye." The presence of this spirit is a strong sign that you can win when fighting or sparring. In daily life, if you hear a person say, "I can't do it," you can see that his or her eyes are dull and have no spirit. On the other hand, if you hear a person saying, "Yes, I can do it," his or her eyes will show power. Such a person has confidence and spirit.

Your mouth should be relaxed, your lips closed, and your tongue loosely touching the upper palate.

3. YOUR SHOULDERS, ARMS, AND HANDS

Your shoulders are down and should be relaxed. In taiji movements where the arm is in the front of the body, the elbows should be relaxed but not pointing straight down toward the floor; they should be at about forty-five degrees to the floor from the body. If you elevate your elbows or shoulders, you create tension in your arms and shoulder area. If you have tension, your energy does not move through the whole system the way it should, and your practice becomes less effective. People find themselves tensed up in many situations: working, planning, cooking, reading, doing computer work, teaching, writing, and even talking. Everyday tension creates energy blockages in your body and reduces both qi and blood circulation. When this happens over a long time, you get headaches, dizziness, insomnia, sinus pressure, low energy, stiffness, infection, emotional problems, anxiety, and tightness in the neck, shoulders, and back. This is when your doctor tries to find a diagnosis for you. Probably 90 percent of doctor's visits are for ailments caused by stress. Physical tension comes from mental tension. The mental tension is from not engaging in the practice of letting go. Taiji practice helps you to let go, remove mental tension, and therefore alleviate physical tension. Proper taiji posture helps you bring awareness to your tension so that you can relieve it. This gives us plenty of reasons to learn to perform taiji correctly.

From a martial arts standpoint, relaxing your shoulders and dropping the elbows is a protective strategy. If your shoulders are raised, your elbows will also be lifted, giving your opponent the chance to take you down or lock you up. Only if you are relaxed are you able to respond quickly to any movement toward you from your opponent.

Your arm should follow your body in every taiji movement. You do not intentionally move your arm but rather let the arm go wherever the body goes. If you focus too much on your arm work, you look like you are dancing rather than doing taiji. This happens to many beginning students. Taiji looks like a form of slow dancing with circular movement of the arms. But the real movement is internal and invisible. When you move the body with full intention, sometimes you can feel the internal moving of the qi. When that happens, you know you are doing it right. The arm movements are minimal and follow the body; the arms only appear to have a big role.

Your wrists should be relaxed and flexible but well controlled. Relaxed doesn't mean floppy, having no strength, and controlled doesn't mean rigid. This will give you more readiness to change in any way you need to in a fighting situation. Of course, we're not expecting to fight, but we do have push hands practice with its martial applications along with taiji practice. In an emergency, we can protect ourselves.

Wrist rigidness is common for beginners but will get better with practice. Again, the more you are relaxed, the more you are able to let the wrist tension go. Your hands should be relaxed with fingers slightly closed together. Your mind should be focused on your relaxed whole palm, not individual fingers. You can feel the heat in your palms—this is qi.

If you make a fist, it should not be really tight. The top portion of the thumb rests above the first finger joint between the index finger and middle finger.

4. YOUR TORSO AND BACK

Your torso should be relaxed. Relaxing the body allows for a smooth flow of energy. If you are tense, you will create stagnation of energy in your body. All internal organs are located in the torso area, and by having a relaxed torso you relax your back as well. No matter how you move your body, your back should be upright and relaxed. You will be very uncomfortable if your body is twisted or bent. You can get hurt or injured if you practice with the wrong body posture. The lower back should be straight and slightly pushed back; you could even call it a pelvic tilt. It's like tucking the buttocks to allow the lower back to be straight and relaxed. Your kidney is in the lower back area, and by relaxing lower back, your kidney area is also "opened"—free from tension. To keep the kidney area open is very important in taiji and qigong practice, as well as in any Chinese martial arts practice. The waist and hips should be relaxed too. The waist and hips connect upper body and lower body and are the most important parts of the body in taiji practice. The lower back, kidney area, reproductive organ area, lower end part of the spine, hip, and lower abdomen are all in what we call the *dan tian* area. This is where qi is stored. It is the center of your body and affects all other parts of the body. If your waist moves, your entire body moves.

From a martial arts aspect, the waist is your *powerhouse*. When your waist is loose, the power generated from your legs can be easily transmitted to your arms through your waist. Your waist can also generate power that directly moves energy to your hands. If your waist is stiff or tight, the power generated from your legs cannot be transmitted to your hands. Your "powerhouse" will therefore have no power. Ancient taiji masters from China said, "All movements are rooted in the feet, initiated from the leg, controlled by the waist, and expressed through your hands and fingers."

5. YOUR LEGS AND FEET

Your legs should be bent during taiji practice, but you don't have to bend very low. Beginners or seniors can just unlock their knees during practice. Advanced students or younger people with a flexible body and strong legs can bend their knees a little more. It depends on each individual's ability. Having a correct stance is more important than just having a low stance. With each shift of your weight and turning of your waist, you can clearly distinguish between substantial or full and insubstantial or empty yin and yang movement. A simple way to grasp the meaning of substantial or full is put all or most of your weight on one leg—that left is now "substantial" or "full." Your other leg with little or no weight on it is "insubstantial" or "empty." Once you begin to understand the idea of substantial and insubstantial, you will have a centered and balanced feeling, solid and grounded no matter what movements you are performing. If you do not feel balanced, it means you haven't found your center or have not gained the skill of controlling the center.

Your feet are planted on the ground with toes slightly grabbing the ground. You will feel very sturdy when you do this. Movement of the foot is the first step in every movement; other parts follow one after the other in this order: foot, leg, hip, waist, upper arm, forearm, hand. Then repeat this sequence in each movement.

6. YOUR ENTIRE BODY

Once you have relaxed all parts of the body, your entire body is rooted, balanced, and centered, just like a big healthy tree with strong roots that can defend against heavy wind or a storm. With whole-body relaxation, you will feel like your "powerhouse" is in standby mode, ready to generate energy. This is a very important skill to learn in taiji. It also helps you relieve stress, detach from all the junk in your mind, and let go of all tension. Through taiji practice, you will improve your coordination too. One taiji principle is expressed by an ancient master this way: "When there is an upward movement, then there is also a downward movement; when there is a left movement, then there is also a right movement." Your body moves before your arm, your leg moves before your body. Each part of the body follows, one after the other.

If you can relax your whole body, you will be able to focus on the dan tian energy and move that energy any way you wish.

7. YOUR BREATHING

Breathing should be deep and slow, and it should go with the movements and intention. But only advanced students should try to incorporate breath techniques, not beginners because doing so can cause confusion when beginners attempt to pair deep breathing with complicated taiji movements. As you practice for a while and master taiji movements, you can start to pay more attention to your breathing. Generally speaking, you exhale when you direct energy out, and you inhale when you bring energy in. If the movement is going up, you inhale, and if going down, you exhale. If you move hands out, you breathe out; if you move hands in, you breathe in. But there are some exceptions to this rule. For some movements, you will need to follow your intuition. Well-trained taiji teachers can also help you learn how to breathe properly.

Certain movements have different breath patterns, which you will learn in the classroom. You should not be afraid to ask your teacher about breathing or any other movements if you have any doubt. If your teacher cannot answer, she or he may need to do more training to find the answer for you. Teaching is also part of learning.

In the next section, I talk about breathing in some movements, which can be used for reference.

Taiji Basic Movement Requirements

Taiji is a whole-body movement with total coordination. This brings benefits to the entire brain. The intuitive part of the brain is activated from whole-body coordination. Recall the principle we discussed above: "Whenever there is movement, the whole body moves. When one part of your body moves, all other parts follow."

Another principle governing taiji movement is that "there is motion in stillness and there is stillness in motion" in every movement. When you move, you feel calm and peaceful. When you are practicing taiji, your mind is quiet, peaceful, and calm. You are able to move internal energy.

"All movements are rooted in the feet, initiated from the leg, controlled by the waist, and expressed through your hands and fingers." We saw this principle above. Again, being rooted through the feet creates a strong root of energy like a strong tree. When your leg starts to move, the waist and then arm follow. This is how it appears in movement. But in reality, once you are rooted, your next focus should be moving the dan tian energy, which is located in the area of the lower abdomen. Many people put too much focus on the hands and arms. In doing so, the body does not generate energy. It causes too much tension and leaves out the center. This will not help your energy flow.

"The mind produces internal movement, and internal movement produces external movement." All movements are directed from your mind. If your mind is not there, your movements do not mean anything, and your taiji is powerless. That is why the mind is the most important part of the practice. Just like anything else, if your mind is off track, you make mistakes when performing tasks.

"The upper and lower parts of the body are coordinated, left and right are coordinated, mind and body are coordinated, and breathing and movements are coordinated."

Do not worry if you feel you have poor coordination; your coordination will improve after practicing for a while.

"All movements are in a circular and continuous motion." There are many things in the natural and physical world that are in the shape of a circle, such as the earth and other heavenly bodies, their motion through the heavens, the eye, many fruits and vegetables, and so many others. Even electricity flow has to be a complete circuit with no breaks. Many of the circles have energy. This is part of the reason why the circular motion is so important in taiji practice. Otherwise, you would not feel the flow; you would just feel the movements.

"Relax the mind, sink the shoulders, elbows, and back, sink qi to dan tian." Keep the lower back straight; distinguish yin and yang movements (empty and full). Each yin and yang movement should be completed. The yang movement is followed by the yin movement. The yin movement is followed by the yang movement. When you complete a yang movement, your yin movement starts; when you complete a yin movement, the yang movement starts. Just like everything else, when something reaches one extreme, the opposite begins. The same phenomenon manifests in society too. For example, when our economy gets strong and we become very hotheaded, it will soon slow down, and stock prices begin to fall. When our economy gets weak, we work harder, and then everything begins to improve. This is a part of Daoist philosophy: events move in a spontaneous flow.

Your weight is continually shifting from left to right, right to left. The weight is 60 percent on one leg and 40 percent on the other; then the movement changes to the opposite and is 60 percent on the other and 40 percent on the first. For younger people, the weight distribution in the shifting can be 70/30. Shifting of weight is constant and continually changing from side to side. The waist position is also constant and continues turning from side to side. This clearly describes the yin and yang of taiji movements.

Taiji Practice Requirements

Although you can practice any way you want, the best way to practice taiji or qigong is in a group. It does not matter how big the group is; what does matter is if the group energy is together or in sync when everyone goes the same speed and same direction. In old Chinese tradition, the group energy is very often emphasized.

In ancient Chinese healing, each individual has energy channels. If the channels are open in one person, it affects another person in the same room. If the channels are open in many individuals, the energy in the room can really be felt. If one person's channels are open and another person's are not, sooner or later that person's channel will be opened as the practice proceeds. You can feel the energy when you practice with a person who has a high energy level and smooth flow of energy through his or her channels. Our students always feel good after practicing taiji in the classroom with other people.

Sometimes you may also be able to tell when someone has too much negative energy. It makes you want to avoid them. But if this person continues to practice taiji or qigong faithfully, his or her energy may change, and you may feel the difference after a while. I have seen this happen in many students. This brings up an idea I would like to express: People *do* change and people *can* change.

Practicing individually is also important. This may be challenging in the beginning especially when you cannot remember the movements. You may be frustrated and sometimes even want to quit. But if you can focus on one movement and repeat it over and over, your body will remember. There are several things to keep in mind that will help you achieve your goal:

- Discipline

- Patience

- Confidence

- Positive attitude

- Diligence

DISCIPLINE

Developing taiji discipline is very important in taiji practice. It is not easy. It takes effort and mind power. Unlike other exercises such as walking, weightlifting, and running on a treadmill, you don't need memory to walk, to lift weights, or use a treadmill. These are all external body workouts not necessarily involving the mind. Taiji and qigong are different. It takes a special person to practice them. Why? First, it is an internal workout where the effort required cannot be seen. Most people, when they learn how much effort is involved, won't take up the challenge. Second, it takes time to learn and practice. Not many people are willing to take the time to learn something difficult that has no monetary reward. Third, it is not a mainstream exercise, so most people go with the crowd and do what other people do. Fourth, the majority of people like to do things fast, not slow. They feel that doing things slowly is a waste of time. Last, the majority of people don't have discipline. Only special people have discipline.

PATIENCE

Nothing comes easily. Nothing comes overnight. Being frustrated can only get you down and make you uncomfortable. Learning taiji is a journey of natural healing; it takes time. There are no shortcuts to learn taiji or qigong. If you don't get it right this week, maybe you will next week, or the next month, or the next year—it doesn't matter how long it takes. Many people think that learning the form is all there is to taiji study. To learn a taiji form is not that difficult. To learn how to do it correctly *is* difficult. It can take a very long time. The taiji form is not really that important. It just gives you a tool for working with your qi. You can use this tool correctly or incorrectly. The correct way to use this tool is to pursue real taiji skill. The incorrect way to use this tool is to show off taiji moves without building a strong foundation. Showing off will only keep you away from being a good taiji practitioner. If you want to do it the correct way, you should be prepared for a long journey. When it's time to show your taiji skill, your performance of the form will be beautiful and filled with qi. If you want to see the breathtaking view from the top of a mountain, you have to plan a trip and make the hike. This can be hard work, but there is a great payoff that makes it worthwhile. Many taiji masters in China have studied for a lifetime and still practice regularly. In Chinese martial arts, there are no belts awarded. The reward is inside the practitioner. When it is time for a real fight or competitive tournament, you can see their genuine skills.

Some people look for shortcuts to success. However, there are no shortcuts. Just like anything else in life, hard work and a solid foundation will allow you to reach higher levels of achievement and build a better character. Trying to find a shortcut is shallow, superficial, and doesn't let us solve real problems. Only real skills acquired through learning and practicing can solve real problems. In the beginning of my teaching, I went to Beijing to be mentored by Master Feng Zhi Qiang. I thought I did well performing in front of Master Feng. But all he said to me was "Too tight, too tight."

That was a big lesson for me. After that, I really began to focus on relaxation in my practice. I can feel the benefits. I also realized that relaxation must come from within.

CONFIDENCE

You must have confidence in yourself. No one is born with skill. But it is really true that you can do anything if you put your mind to it. People have different strengths and weaknesses—nobody is perfect. Everyone has different experience. Some people learn certain things more quickly than others. However, everyone can learn if they choose to, have enough determination, and engage their mind fully in the learning process. Just like when you go to college, you will graduate if you choose to graduate—and you will drop out if you choose to drop out. If you commit to using taiji to enrich your life, stay healthy, create a harmonious life, and learn the science of human energy, you will learn it very well. Even though you may feel uncoordinated in the beginning, sooner or later you will feel much better. Your confidence will increase each day.

POSITIVE ATTITUDE

A positive attitude is important for everything. You will not succeed if you have a negative attitude. This is also true of taiji. You may choose to do some other physical activity or exercise, which can also give you benefits. With anything you want to learn, you should always keep a positive attitude. Sometimes you might have a negative experience, but this is no reason to be negative.

I asked a patient to study taiji for stress relief. She tried one class and said she hated it. It was a very negative thing to say. I asked her why she hated taiji, and she responded that the instructor made her uncomfortable. She did not think she could learn taiji, so she quit. After I explained what taiji is and how to practice, she decided to try again and did much better.

DILIGENCE

Like everything else in life, practice makes perfect. Learning taiji is the same: without diligent practice, you will not develop taiji skill or reach higher levels. A doctor graduated from medical school and got his license, then started his medical practice. Another doctor has been practicing medicine for more than ten years. Who would you choose to be your doctor? What if you need a service from a company—would you choose a new company or a well-known company that has been providing the service for many years? Remember, good skill comes from diligent practice. The practice of taiji should be fun, not a chore. If you think it is fun, you will practice regularly. If you think it is work, you may not do it.

Taiji Mental Requirements

- Full concentration
- Awareness of energy center and surroundings
- Relaxation
- Noncompetitiveness
- Modesty

Full Concentration

We have mentioned before that learning taiji requires your full concentration. Leave everything behind, detach from all things, and cherish your precious time with taiji, and it will make you feel great. If your mind starts to wander, you should simply refocus. We call taiji "moving meditation" because it involves full concentration. This way you feel like you cleanse your mind during your practice. You focus on the middle part of the body and let the other parts of the body move naturally.

Awareness of Energy Center and Surroundings

You need to be aware of your energy center and surroundings. Finding your energy center and focusing on it helps you to be rooted. Once you know how to move your core energy in your energy center, no matter how you move your body, other parts of the body always follow. The energy center is in the lower abdomen. As we've said, we call it the dan tian. This is the middle part of the body, connecting the body's upper and lower parts. It is adjacent to your hip, supported by your kidney qi, and managed by your mind. You need to know how to use your hips to guide the other parts of the body. Be aware that you may move the hips the wrong way, thereby misleading the other parts of the body. But you can feel when you move the hips the wrong way. The way of self-correction is to move the way your body feels comfortable.

You also need to be aware of your surroundings. Don't necessarily let your attention be fixed on just one thing. This way you know what is going on in your space, and you can control your energy and movement. This is especially important when you use your taiji skills for self-defense.

Relaxation

I keep talking about relaxation. In my experience, people know this word but don't know how to actually relax. In my years of teaching, I have probably repeated this word several thousand times.

Your body and mind must be relaxed. There should be no tension in any part of your body. Taiji is a simple yet sophisticated technique for relaxation. Let your muscles be free of tension and your mind free of worry and empty of thoughts. Let your qi blend into the universe. This allows your energy to flow smoothly, your mind to be decluttered, and a maximum relaxation response to be produced. Relaxation allows you to really enjoy the taiji movements. That is how taiji works. You should not be stressed during your practice, even if you are corrected many times and still cannot remember how to do it. It is no big deal; just go with the flow.

If any parts of the body feel tight, you need to stop and start again with complete relaxation. Don't be afraid to stop and start again.

Noncompetitiveness

There is no competition in taiji practice. There is no need for you to compare your skill to other people's skill. Taiji is for health, healing, and prevention; building inner peace; stress relief; and delaying the aging process. Don't worry if someone's coordination is better than yours. We all have different strengths and weaknesses. This is completely normal. Only compete with yourself to improve day by day; do not compete with other people. There are no belts in taiji. The real belt is measured by how you have improved the overall health of your mind, body, and spirit and how you have improved in relaxation, coordination, health, and happiness.

I used to be competitive, but from years of learning, I realized that life is not about competition. You only compete with yourself, not with others. This allows you to improve. Life is about learning and contributing, putting out 100 percent of your effort. Life is also about balance: you work and you relax, you learn and you do by putting theory into practice. You make time for your friends or other people and then you make time for yourself. Most importantly, you love yourself and you love others.

Modesty

Learning taiji is a journey that may not be easy for some people. It has many components. You should not think you have learned enough after learning a taiji form or even multiple forms. Some people think learning a taiji form is all they need to know about taiji. Taiji is much more involved than just a form or a way to get regular exercise. On your taiji journey, you will learn new things and improve your skill year after year. Taiji involves so many things: meditation, martial arts, healing, disease prevention, Daoist philosophy, and Chinese medicine. My own experience had proved to me that taiji has healing benefits when practiced correctly. When I was teaching, I practiced less. Now I not only practice more but practice more in depth. I realized that doing taiji slower helps my hip by strengthening it. My hip pain reduced. It also helps my balance a great deal.

If you are modest, your instructor will teach you as much as he or she knows. However, if you think you have learned enough, the instructor will stop sharing with you because you have closed the door to learning. Besides studying taiji, you should be familiar with Daoist philosophy. In bookstores you can find a copy of the *Tao Te Ching* (or *Daodejing*). Just read one chapter each night, and you will accumulate wisdom. When you have acquired this knowledge, you will gain the ability to solve many problems in life. Understanding the Dao helps bring wisdom to all you do.

How to Avoid Injuries in Taiji Practice

In general, the practice of taiji and qigong is safe. I have not heard of any negative effects on people's health. But it could cause injury if done the wrong way, just like anything else. If you turn your body incorrectly, you could hurt your back or neck. If you bend and raise your body improperly, you could hurt your back. Here are some tips to avoiding injury.

1. BEGINNERS AND OLDER PEOPLE SHOULD AVOID A LOW STANCE

If you are a beginning student or just starting to learn taiji, you have not yet developed leg strength. If you try too hard to do a low stance (see YouTube for many examples of martial artists using this stance), your muscles and joints may be injured. Keep in mind, some of the martial artists started at a very young age and some are professionals. Some of them had a martial arts major in college, and some were on a martial arts team and competed at high levels. They had much more practice than regular people. Their bodies had prepared for this kind of practice for a long time. You should practice taiji in a comfortable stance. After you have studied and practiced for a while, you automatically lower your stance without trying because your qi and leg muscles are stronger. It happens spontaneously and naturally as time goes by. It is not wise to compete with others who have a low stance. Also, from a preventive health point of view, a low stance could possibly cause injuries, which has happened to many martial art practitioners. This is why they do qigong when they are getting older; they are trying to heal their body.

2. BEGINNERS SHOULD NOT WORRY ABOUT "PERFECTION"

Taiji is not about the "perfection of movement," though we want our students to learn well and to follow taiji principles. When first learning taiji, your muscles, ligaments, and the soft tissue surrounding the joints are not as flexible. Trying too hard can cause discomfort, fatigue, or injury and can block energy flow in the body.

Beginners should not try to do everything "right" but just get used to the movements and flowing energy. Focus on the body motion of shifting and turning, not on detailed movements, especially arms movements. Taiji is a multidimensional practice, and it takes time to learn it well. After you study taiji for a while and have learned the form, you then can start making corrections. My best suggestion: go with the flow. This is real Daoist practice.

3. GRADUALLY INCREASE THE TIME OF PRACTICE

In the beginning, you don't have to work very hard. If you practice by yourself, you can practice fifteen to forty-five minutes per day. Each month, you can increase the length of time you practice. With explanation, warm-up exercises, and qigong, a taiji class normally takes one hour, although some classes may be longer. The optimum time for practice is forty-five minutes to one hour per day, with some warm-up. If you have learned several forms of taiji (such as Chen style, combined style, or taiji sword)— or qigong or other martial arts—you can practice one and a half hours each time or daily. For advanced students, one and a half hours to two hours is ideal. The advanced practitioner may incorporate other internal martial arts such as bagua or xingyi.

4. ALTERNATE THE PRACTICE OF STATIONARY MOVEMENTS AND WALKING MOVEMENTS

When I say stationary movements, I mean movements performed without changing your location on the ground. Stationary movement is involved in qigong, taiji basics, and taiji movement without walking (as in the taiji thirteen steps or poses). Alternating between stationary and walking practice will give you balanced training and help you keep your attention focused.

5. ALWAYS WARM UP BEFORE PRACTICE; SLOWLY COOL DOWN AFTERWARD

You can choose any kind of warm-up exercise. You can power walk, stretch, jump rope, or anything else that will help get your blood flowing. In this book I provide some warm-up exercises to help promote circulation. After practice, you should not immediately sit down for a long time. You should let the muscles slowly cool down. If the muscles are warm and then suddenly become cool for a long period, it causes stagnation of the qi and blood circulation as well as muscle stiffness. Some athletes have muscle stiffness and chronic inflammation of the soft tissue due to improper cooldown. Follow this simple sequence: warm-up exercise (including light stretching), qigong, taiji, and stretching—or add some qigong.

6. CAUTIONS ABOUT CERTAIN ILLNESSES

If you have arthritis in your knees, you should keep your stance higher by just slightly bending your knees and trying to be comfortable. If you have balancing issues, you can slow the movements down to try to restore your balance. If you have some inflammation in a certain joint that prohibits you from moving that joint, you can modify the movement. If you have heart disease, you can pay more attention to your breathing, which you can learn from your instructor. If you feel short of breath or are having palpitations, you should slow down or take a short break. You should always listen to your body and never force yourself to continue practicing if you are uncomfortable. It takes time to build good qi and blood circulation. If you have poor energy, you will need to practice regularly every day. Start with fifteen to twenty minutes a day for the first week, with five minutes of warm-up. Then increase to thirty minutes a day. You can practice two times a day, thirty minutes each time, if you wish. Once you get used to this pattern, you can gradually increase the time.

Suggestions and Precautions for Your Practice

1. YOUR BELIEF AND TRUST

If you don't believe in taiji and qigong even after trying a class, there is nothing wrong with that. Taiji is not for everyone, same as anything else: some people like it very much, and others don't care for it. However, some people have changed their minds after persisting and getting good results. It's just a matter of finding a form of exercise that suits your temperament. Any negative feeling will not bring good results. It is like anything else in life—do what you believe in and what you are attracted to.

2. MORNING PRACTICE

Some people feel sluggish, stiff, or like they have low energy in the morning. If this describes you, do some simple qigong, stretching, and other movement to get your energy flowing. For this purpose, I offer here a short form called Morning Routine. See chapter 4 for more detailed explanations of horse ride pushing palm, bending forward, and knock the body.

1. Open to see the sky: take a deep breath and raise arms in front of the body and then all the way up over your head. Breathe out and move arms outward to the sides and then downward. Repeat this eight times.

2. Horse ride pushing palm: in a horse stance (knees are unlocked, back is relaxed), palms facing forward, suddenly push one palm with a fast exhalation, then fast push the other palm with the quick exhalation. Repeat eight times. (For detailed instructions on horse stance, see "Taiji Basics" in the "Foundation Practice" section in chapter 4.)

3. Bending forward: take a deep breath, raise hands and arms up over your head, exhale lowering your upper body, bending forward until your hands reach

as low as possible, maybe touching the floor. At the same time, relax and breathe.

4. Knock the body: using either your palm or fist, knock the body from the shoulder downward toward the hand, then the lower back, and down your legs. The "knock" is not hard. It's more of a pat.

5. Take a deep, slow breath to end this short routine.

If you practice early in the morning, you should not feel hungry or thirsty. Drinking a little water before your morning practice helps cleanse the body. Eat a piece of fruit or something else small. It is better to practice before breakfast. But there is nothing wrong with practicing after breakfast as long as you allow at least one hour after eating.

3. SETTING A TIME FOR YOUR PRACTICE

When you set a time to practice, make sure you have this time for yourself and won't be interrupted. This allows you to focus completely and produce maximum energy. If you are interrupted, your energy is interrupted. This explains why taiji students get more benefits than their instructors. Instructors must focus on teaching, which interrupts their own inner practice. For this reason, some students are more energized than the instructor after a class.

4. DIRECTION AND LOCATION FOR INDIVIDUAL PRACTICE

Chinese tradition says females should face south and males should face north. This might be related to the magnetic energy of the atmosphere. However, in modern life, we don't need to follow this tradition, and it is not practical anyway. For instance, if you are in a classroom, you need to face the direction the teacher instructs. If you practice by yourself, just follow your intuition and choose the direction that makes you feel good, tranquil, and peaceful. This will be the right direction for you. For outdoor practice, find a good natural setting—under a tree, near a garden, next to a pond, on a big lawn, or at a park. I always encourage people to practice outdoors to get more fresh air and natural beauty. I tried one night doing qigong at a park when there was a full moon. Several students went with me, and it was very special. We had a really good time, and it felt like we were on a different planet.

5. FREQUENCY OF PRACTICE

I recommend that you practice daily, even just fifteen minutes if you are short of time. Then on the weekend when you do have some time, you can practice for sixty minutes or more. If you really don't have time, practicing three to five times a week is still good. You don't need to feel bad if you miss practicing once or twice. As long as you have good intentions, you can always keep up your practice. Some people find that they miss practicing taiji when they skip several sessions. This is a good sign. We call this a healthy craving—your body misses the energy boost that comes from taiji. This is a good sign because it means you'll have a tendency to do things that are healthy for you.

In my own case, my legs hurt more if I don't practice. This makes me aware of my need for daily practice.

6. KEEPING WHOLESOME AIR IN YOUR PRACTICE AREA

Do not practice if the air in the room is not good. An odor—like a moldy or chemical smell—can be distracting. You pay more attention to the bad smell than to the practice. Some odors stimulate the central nervous system and can cause headache, nausea, dizziness, light-headedness, or other symptoms. In this case, you need to change the location of your practice or just go outside.

7. OUTDOOR PRACTICE

If you practice outdoors, which I highly recommend, you should avoid heavy winds and extreme cold or hot temperatures. Heavy winds and extreme temperatures distract your attention and affect energy flow in the body. Extreme cold weather affects blood flow (unless you are jogging) and makes it hard to produce good energy. In traditional Chinese medicine, extreme cold is one of the evils that cause illness. If it is too hot, you could be dehydrated or suffer a heat stroke. But if your body tends to be cold and you like hot weather, make sure to have plenty of water available if you choose to practice outdoors.

8. EMPTYING YOUR SYSTEM

You should relieve your bowel and bladder before your practice. Waste contains toxins and should not be retained. Doing so causes an energy blockage, which may render your workout ineffective.

9. WHEN YOU ARE EITHER TOO HUNGRY OR OVERFULL

If you are too hungry, practice can deplete your energy or make you tired instead of energized. Some people may have low blood sugar levels, and not eating can cause light-headedness, dizziness, and nausea. If you are overfull, on the other hand, you already have a blockage in the middle part of the body. It can be uncomfortable and sometimes cause cramps in your stomach. That is why I recommend having a snack before practice. Always carrying some healthy snacks is a good habit.

10. GOOD QUALITY SLEEP AS AID TO HEALING AND PRACTICE

A good night's sleep is important in Chinese healing systems. Quality sleep indicates balanced organ energy. Getting a good night's sleep makes a big difference in your energy level when practicing taiji.

If you have slight insomnia, taiji practice can help you. If you have severe insomnia, you need to check with your doctor to find out why and get some help. In most cases, the insomnia is caused by stress. Learning Daoist philosophy can help you to manage your stress and understand the laws of nature. Severe insomnia can affect your energy and make the practice less effective.

11. IMPORTANCE OF COTTON AND OTHER SOFT CLOTHES AND SHOES

As a natural energy practice, taiji comes from nature. We try to harmonize with nature in both thought and action. One simple way to be more in tune with nature is by wearing clothes and shoes made from natural fabrics, like cotton. Cotton is more comfortable than synthetics. You can easily notice the difference. Cotton also helps absorb sweat. Never wear high heels when you practice taiji. Also avoid wearing a hat when practicing taiji or qigong. When you are bending forward (as in some qigong forms), or outdoors where there is wind, your hat will fall on the ground. Some qigong forms also involve self-massage, which includes massaging the head. It is better if the head is uncovered to get maximum benefits from self-massage.

12. WHEN YOU ARE SICK

If you have a slight cold, you can still practice, and you most likely will feel better afterward. But if you have a severe cold or flu, it is better to rest and not risk depleting your energy. The best way is to listen to your body and take a good rest if needed. This will allow your body to heal faster. Overstressing your body will do it more harm. During resting periods, you can still do qigong breathing, which helps the healing process.

13. AVOIDING ALCOHOL AND OTHER SUBSTANCES

Taiji students and practitioners do not use substances that abuse the body. Our purpose is to nourish our body, not to abuse it. On occasion we can drink socially. We sometimes go out with friends and family for a dinner gathering and consume a little alcohol. This is acceptable if you have just a few drinks. On nights like this, you can enjoy the company of friends and not have to think about training taiji. Alcohol disperses your energy and affects your brain's chemistry. You sometimes notice that your balance is off and your energy scattered after drinking.

14. MODERATION IN SEX

In Daoist practice, everything needs to be in moderation, including sex. The principle is not "the more the better." Too much sex depletes your kidney energy, especially in men. In Chinese medicine, the kidney energy is very important in human health and longevity. Kidney energy is like the "backbone" of all organs and supports all organs. If your kidney energy is weak, you may have back pain, reproductive organ malfunction, impotence, arthritis, early gray hairs, dental problems, poor memory, and low energy. These are also signs of aging.

15. HEALTHY DIET

Taiji practitioners should always have a healthy diet. Eating small meals with lots of vegetables is an ideal healthy diet. Eat less meat and fewer carbs, and increase your vegetable and fruit intake. I disagree with a purely vegetarian diet such as vegan diets. Pure vegetarian diets have limited food choices in the United States, and some people suffer from imbalanced nutrition and develop illnesses. In Asia and some Middle Eastern countries, there are many more food choices for the vegetarian diet. I believe if your diet is varied and moderate, you should have no diet-related problems. Eating every kind of food provides you with all necessary nutrients. I had a twenty-year-old patient who got sick several years after eliminating meat from her diet. She became anemic, fatigued, and suffered hair loss. She sought help from her primary care doctor who recommended that she eat red meat to help her low blood count. Unfortunately, after eating no meat for several years, this patient's digestive gland stopped producing enzymes for breaking down meat. She developed severe digestive problems after adding meat into her diet. It took me a while to help her to restore her digestive health.

If you grow up with a diet you cannot change, or if you have religious reasons to keep a certain diet, just eat following your belief system. If something goes wrong due to your diet, you can either accept your condition or make some changes to improve your health. Keep in mind that things can always change and that there is nothing wrong with change.

Guidelines for Your Learning Journey

If you are a beginner, I am here to provide you with some guidelines for learning, to be used over ten weeks. These guidelines apply whether your learning takes place in the classroom or by yourself. If you are a taiji teacher with beginner-level students, you can also use these guidelines to help them. And if you are an advanced student, I assume you have already developed your own sequence of practice. But if you haven't, I recommend you follow this sequence: *warm-up exercise*, *foundation practice*, *qi practice*, *form practice*, *stretching*, and *cooldown*.

Learning taiji is easier with a structured approach. It's like having a business plan. Learning taiji should also have a plan, which is why I am writing this book to help people learn taiji effectively. There are several steps when you practice taiji:

1. Warm-up exercise: to avoid injuries. There are three layers of warm-up:
   - Gentle warm-up to start
   - Light cardio to get the blood flowing
   - Stretching to release muscle tension

2. Foundation practice: to get practice in applying taiji principles, build a taiji foundation, and build better qi. This is the beginning of qi practice. There are several forms of foundation practice:
   - Taiji basics
   - Taiji qigong
   - Taiji thirteen movements
   - Cat walk (taiji walk)

3. Form practice: to move the qi. Whichever form you are learning—such as Yang style, Chen style, or Wu style—will be fine. Choose a short form to start if you are a beginner. If you have been doing taiji for a while, you can choose a longer form. I prefer to do a short form multiple times rather than a long form one time.

4. Stretching and cooldown: to end the practice. Everything should have a beginning and an ending. A cooldown technique brings a sense of completion, a feeling of qi coming back to oneself rather than being dispersed.

CHAPTER 4

Taiji Practice Step by Step

Warm-Up Exercise

THE WARM-UP HAS THREE PARTS: gentle warm-up, light cardio, and stretching. The warm-up exercises listed below involve whole-body movements. They are designed to activate energy and blood flow as well as loosen the muscles, tendons, and joints. They will also help the student avoid injury during taiji practice. This is very important for all practitioners and students. If you want to practice taiji in the morning, warm-up exercises can wake you up better than coffee (though this does not mean you need to quit drinking coffee). You can also use a short-distance run for a warm-up followed by stretching. However, running can be difficult depending on the weather, or if you have problems with your knees or other joints.

To practice the warm-up exercise, you can go through all the movements listed here or just do some of the movements from each category as time and physical ability allow. If you have trouble with certain movements, you can start gently in the beginning and then gradually increase the intensity, or you can skip the movement you have trouble with. You can also choose some warm-up exercise movements before taiji practice and some for after practice. You should especially do stretching before and after. A warm-up exercise can be ten to fifteen minutes depending on the individual. If I don't have much time, I will do seven minutes. If you have more problems in one area, you can spend more time and focus on that area. For instance, if you have back tightness, you can spend more time doing the exercises that help you loosen your back. Each one has its own focus and works on a specific part of the body.

I always like to use music because it provides extra benefits to our health. You can choose whatever music you wish. For warm-up, the music can be faster or uplifting; for taiji practice, the music can be slower and peaceful.

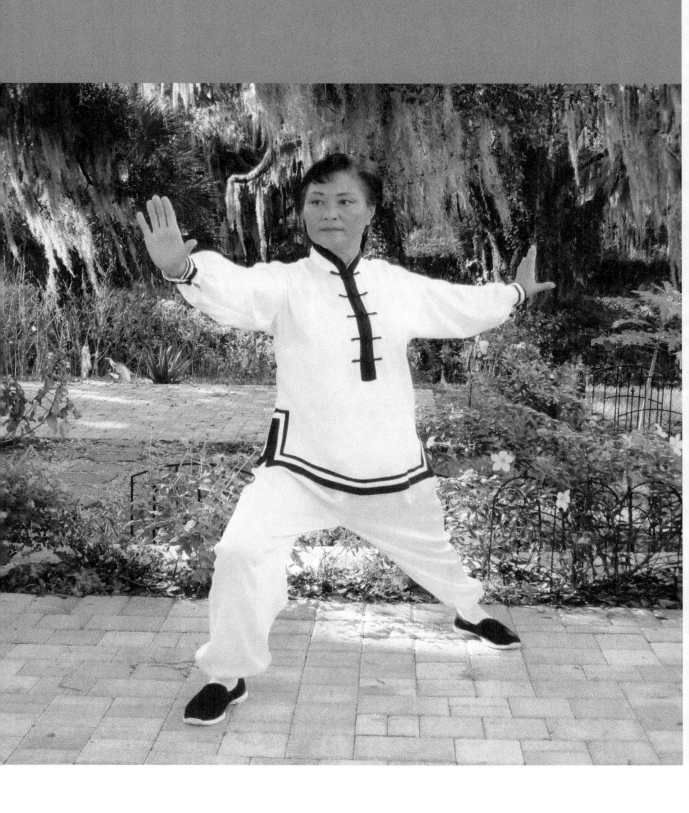

Lifting Heels and Body

- This is an easy movement. Lift your heels to lift your body. You can lift your body two times with each inhalation and two times with each exhalation

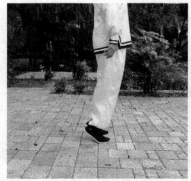

Neck Movement

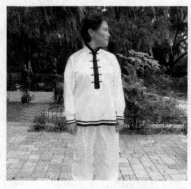
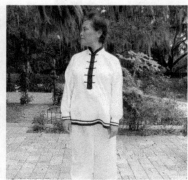

- Always do these movements gently and smoothly, especially if you have neck problems. Turn your head gently and smoothly to the left and then to the right. Do this four times.

- Next move your head up and down four times.

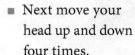
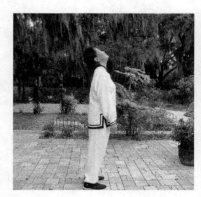
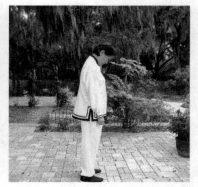

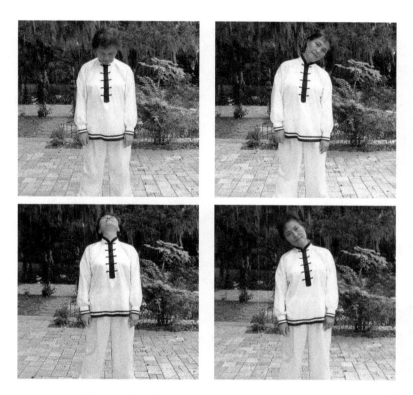

■ Next roll your head in one direction four times and in the other direction four times.

■ Finally, stretch your neck by holding your head down for two breaths.

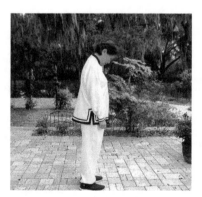

Shoulder Movement

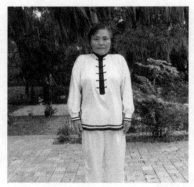

- Move your shoulders up and down. Repeat four times.

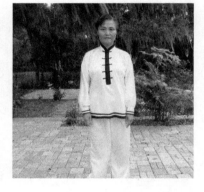

- Rotate your shoulders forward and then backward, four times in each direction.

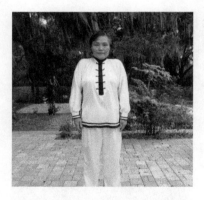

- Then inhale and move shoulders up, exhale, and move shoulders down. Do this four times too.

Circle Arms

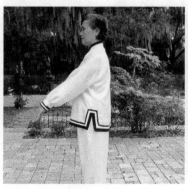
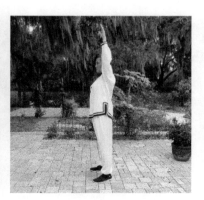

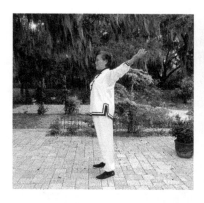 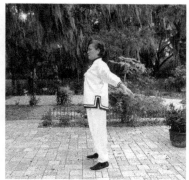

- Circle left arm forward in a big circle four times, then backward four times. Circle the right arm forward four times, then backward four times.

Elbow and Wrist Rotation

- This is not hard to do. Rotate your wrist in one direction and then the other.

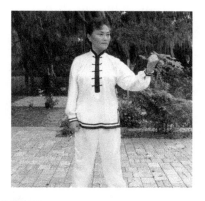

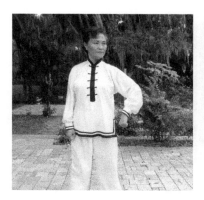 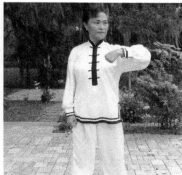

- Next rotate your elbow in one direction, then the other. Do the same rotations on the other arm.

Arm Press: Front, Back, Above Head

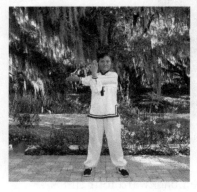

- Use the right forearm to press the left upper arm against your chest. Hold this position for three breaths. Then use the left forearm to press the right upper arm against your chest. Hold this position for three breaths.

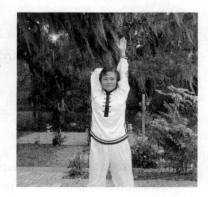

- Next put both your arms over your head and grab your left arm with your right hand. Hold for a breath. Then change sides by simply grabbing your right arm with your left hand. Hold for a breath.

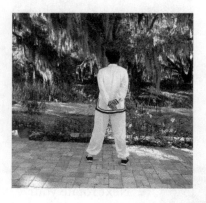

- Use the right hand to grab the left wrist behind the body and hold for a breath. Then use the left hand to grab the right wrist behind the body and hold for a breath. Then repeat once more on each side.

- Use the right hand to grab the left hand over your head. Then bend your body to the right. Stay in this position for two breaths. Change sides and use the left hand to grab the right hand over your head. Then bend your body to the left. Stay in this position for two breaths.

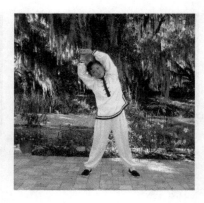

Waist Rotation

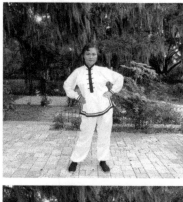 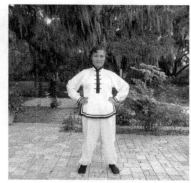

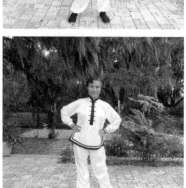 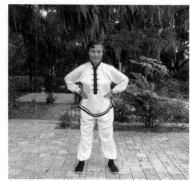

- This is also easy. Circle your hips in one direction eight times, then in the other direction eight times. Breathe normally.

Knee Rotation

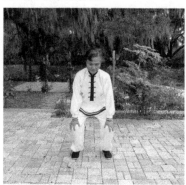 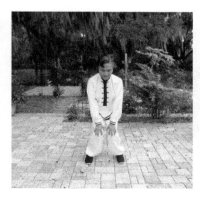

- Feet are shoulder width apart. Circle your knees inward eight times.

- Next circle outward eight times.

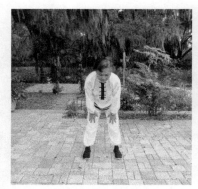 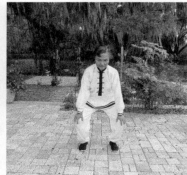

Ankle Rotation

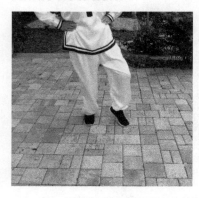

- Put your big toe on the ground in front of you. Circle your foot outward eight times. Then circle your foot inward eight times.

Upper-Body Rotation

- Take a deep breath. Raise your arms above your head.

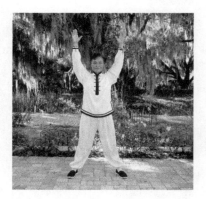

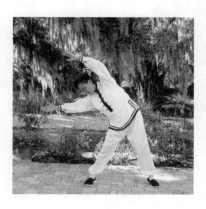

- Exhale and lower your body to the right.

■ Then circle downward.

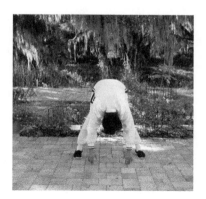

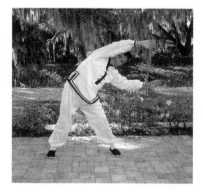

■ Then circle upward toward the left.

■ Then circle upward. Circle four times. Also circle your body in the opposite direction. Lower your body to the left, then downward, then upward to the right, then upward making a big circle. Again, circle four times.

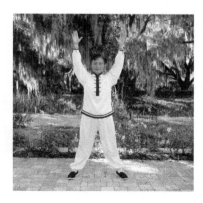

PART II: LIGHT CARDIO

This part involves faster movement than the previous one to get your blood moving. But you should go with your own ability.

Shake Hands

Shake whole hands in any direction. This shaking will get energy moving.

Arm Reaches Opposite

This exercise has both cardio and stretching benefits.

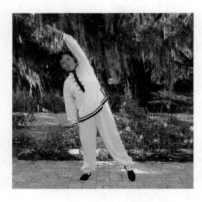

- Reach up and to the right with your left arm. Do this four times.

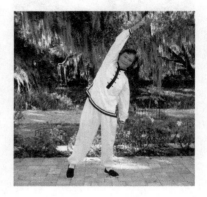

- Next reach up and to the left with your right arm. Do this four times.

Swing Arms While Turning Body

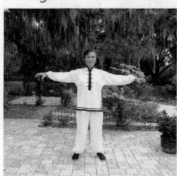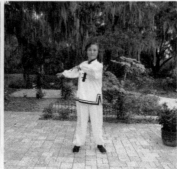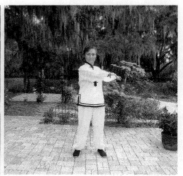

- When you swing your arms while turning your body, allow yourself to relax. You don't need to move your head; this way you get a double benefit. You loosen your spinal vertebrae, and at the same time, your neck area is worked.

Reach Up, Touch Down

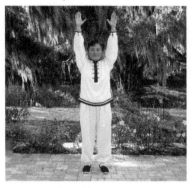

- Inhale while reaching up with your hands.

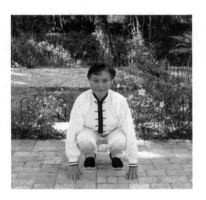

- Exhale while lowering your body and hips until you can touch the floor.
    Repeat this eight times.

Step to Side, Reach Up, Touch Down

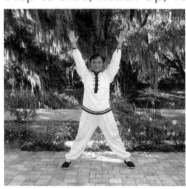

- Step to your left and reach up.

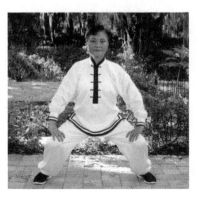

- Bend your knees and exhale as your hands touch your knees.

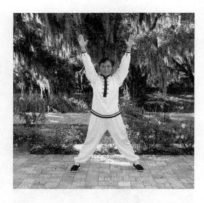

- Inhale and reach up.

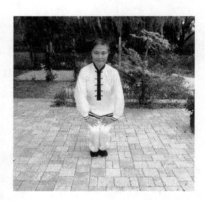

- Exhale as you bring the left foot back next to the right foot. Bend your knees and place your hands on your knees. Come back to standing. Now repeat the movement in the other direction. Step to your right and reach upward. Bend your knees and exhale as your hands touch your knees. Inhale and reach up. Then exhale as your right foot comes back next to your left foot. Bend your knees, and at the same time, your hands touch your knees. Come back to standing. Repeat four times total.

Forward Lunge Push Palm

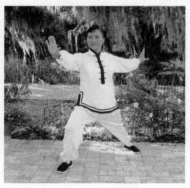

- Step forward with your right foot, and at the same time push your right hand forward and your left hand back, both hands at shoulder level. Then step back and bring your arms back to the front of your chest.

- Step forward with your left foot, and at the same time push your left hand forward and your left hand back, both hands at shoulder level. Step back and bring the arms back to the front of your chest.

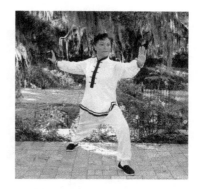

Arm-Elbow-Wrist Rotation while Shifting Weight

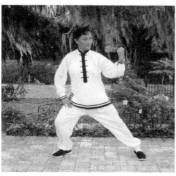 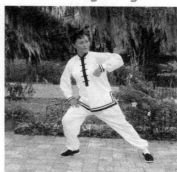

- Shift your weight to your right, and at the same time rotate your left elbow/arm upward.

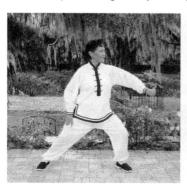 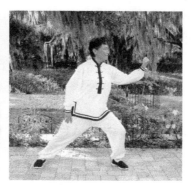

- Then shift your weight to your left, and rotate the elbow and arm downward and end with the fist upward. Repeat this eight times. Next after returning to the initial position, shift your weight to the left, and at the same time rotate the right fist, elbow, and arm upward, then inward. Shift your weight to your right, and rotate right fist, elbow, and arm downward, then upward. Do this eight times again.

Swing Leg

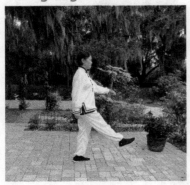 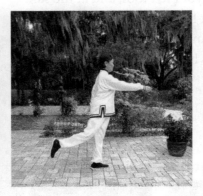

- Put weight on your left leg. Swing your right leg forward and backward fifty times. Put weight on your right leg. Swing your left leg forward and backward fifty times. Make sure to relax your lower back. This warm-up exercise is very good for your lower back, hip, and knee.

Horse Stance Push Palms Forward

It is important to do horse stance correctly. This stance is used in many martial arts and has many benefits, including improved control of your body, increased ability to focus, strengthening of the lower back, an easy way to find your energy center, increased stability of the body, improved brain-body connection, and a more rooted stance.

Here's how to do it.

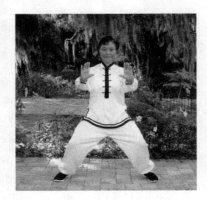

- In a wide stance, take a deep breath, and raise your arms in front of your body, palms pushed out forward. Exhale and sink the body, especially the tailbone, while relaxing the entire back. You can tuck your buttocks forward to open the curve in the lower back area. Sink your arms (elbows) naturally so that your hands are about shoulder level. You should feel very natural in this position.

PART III: STRETCHING

Neck Stretches

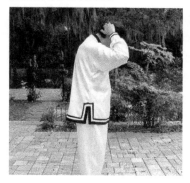

- Use both hands to gently hold your head down for three breaths.

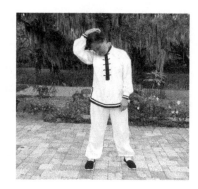

- Turn your head forty-five degrees to the right, and gently hold your head down in this position for three breaths. Repeat on the left side.

Forward Lunge

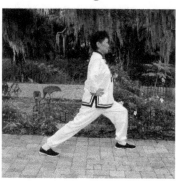

- Step forward with your left foot, slightly off your centerline. Put 70 percent of your weight on your left leg, and hold this position for three breaths. Step back.

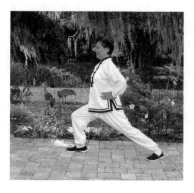

- Step forward with your right foot slightly off your centerline. Put 70 percent of your weight on your right leg, and hold this position for three breaths. Step back. Repeat one more time on both sides.

Side Lunge

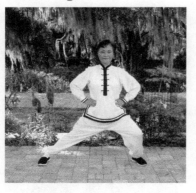

- Take a big step to your left. Put 70 percent of your weight on your left leg, and hold this position for three breaths. Step back.

  Repeat on the right side. Take a big step to your right. Put 70 percent of your weight on your right leg, and hold this position for three breaths. Step back.

Side Stretching

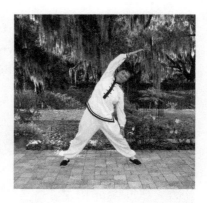

- Stand with your feet apart, about one and half times your shoulder width. Raise your right arm above your head, and lean to the left. Hold this position for three breaths.

  Repeat on the opposite side. Raise your left arm above your head, and lean to the right. Hold this position for three breaths.

Hug Knee

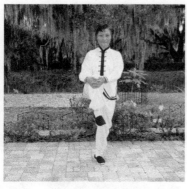

- Hold right knee up with both hands in front of the body. Stay for three breaths.

  Repeat with the left knee.

Hold Ankle with Opposite Hand

- Grab your left ankle with your right hand. Hold this position for three breaths.
  Repeat with the right ankle.

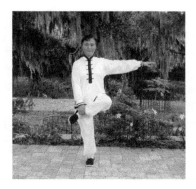

Stretch Quadriceps

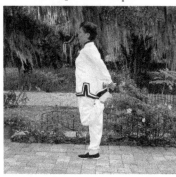

- Hold your left foot behind your buttock, and hold this position for three breaths.
  Repeat with your right foot.

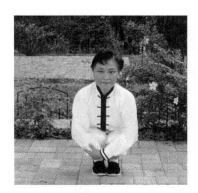

Squat Hugging Knees

- Raise your hips (buttocks), lower your head, and relax. Try to keep your feet flat on the ground. If this is uncomfortable, you can lift your heels as needed.

Crossed-Leg Squat

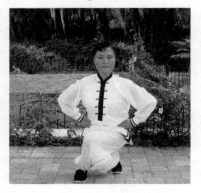

- Cross your left foot in front of your right foot. Exhale and sink the body into a crossed-leg squat with your right knee crossed behind your left knee. The heel of the right foot is lifted. Stay in this position for a breath or two. Inhale, raising the body slowly. Exhale and return your feet to the normal position.

    Now perform the same movement on the other side. Cross your right foot in front of your left foot. Exhale, sink the body, and complete the movement as above.

Stretch Hamstring

- Hold your right toe with your right hand, and use your left hand to support the leg. Hold this position for a breath or two.
  Repeat with the left leg.

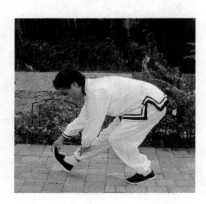

Bending Forward

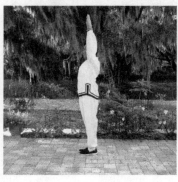

- Reach upward with both hands. Inhale.

- Bend forward at the hip, and relax the torso and neck. Hold this position for a few breaths, then return to your starting position.

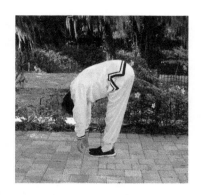

Knocking the Body

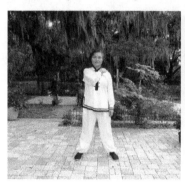

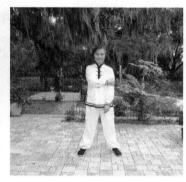

- Use either your fists or palms to knock (pat) your body. Knock your left arm from the shoulder downward.

- Then knock from the right shoulder and down the right arm.

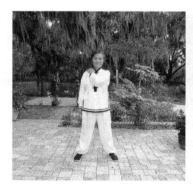

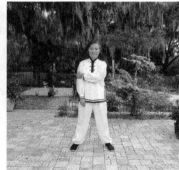

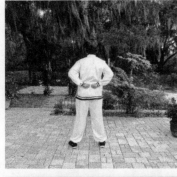

■ Knock your lower back.

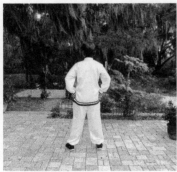
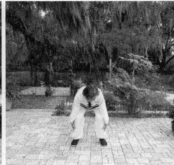
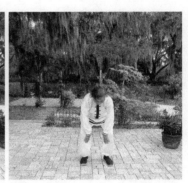

■ Then knock your hips and legs.

Foundation Practice

FOUNDATION PRACTICE INVOLVES PUTTING the taiji principles into practice in taiji walking, taiji basics, taiji qigong, and taiji thirteen movements.

Understanding the foundation of taiji is very important in your practice. Without basic training, your learning could take a long time, and your taiji form may produce less qi. You will not get the benefits you want. It is like building a house: without a strong foundation, the house will not be strong. Many people focus only on the taiji form or taiji movements and may not achieve good qi, good balance, a clear mind, and healing benefits. They have only the taiji frame but no core, no contents. The frame is weak without content just like a house with no people and no furniture.

You will notice in foundation practice that there are a lot of circles. This is to get you to be more familiar with circular movement, which is one of the characteristics of taiji movements. You will also notice there are some repeated movements; no matter how many are repeated, just do it because you will get better and better at those movements with each repetition.

There is no hard-and-fast rule about how many times you should perform a movement. But with my students, I like to use the rule of the "magical five," which is simply to do an exercise at least five times once you know how to perform it correctly. Five repetitions are adequate for getting the full benefit of the exercise and also for locking knowledge of how to perform the technique into muscle memory. So unless instructed otherwise, do each exercise at least five times.

During foundation practice, you can either do them all or choose a selection to practice if you are short on time. The key is daily practice. If you can invite someone to join you, your practice will be more effective. Practicing with a partner is not only motivating, but as we said above, group practice generates a lot of qi.

Part 1: Taiji Basics (Exercise Sequence)

1. SHIFTING WEIGHT SIDE TO SIDE

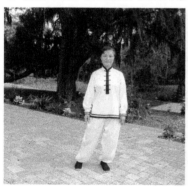 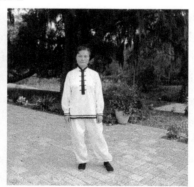

■ This exercise is not difficult. Stand in horse stance, feet one and a half shoulder width apart. Unlock your knees, put 70 percent to 80 percent of your weight onto one leg, then move weight to the other leg, shifting right to left and left to right ten to twenty times until you feel more relaxed, especially your lower back.

2. SHIFTING AND TURNING

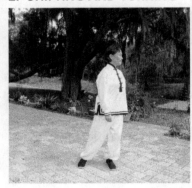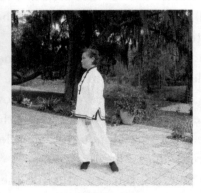

- This is a multidimensional movement. Because you know how to shift your weight, all you need to do is turn to the side you have the weight on. Then move your weight to the other side while turning to the other side. Repeat the shifting and turning practice. This is very important and should not be ignored.

3. LEFT HAND CIRCLES OUTWARD, THEN CIRCLES INWARD

Because you have done the above practice of shifting and turning, all you need is to add your arm and hand work. Because you are turning, it looks like you are moving your left hand down, then to the right. But this is a misconception. That is why many people who learn from a video cannot get this detail.

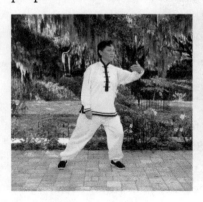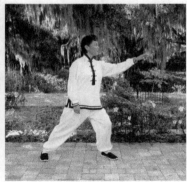

- Shift your weight to the left. Then allow your left arm to naturally circle from the lower dan tian (lower abdomen) upward, then outward, palm facing upward.

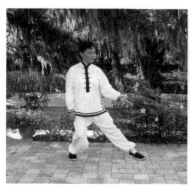 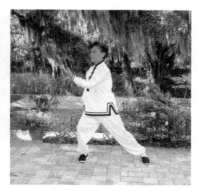

■ Next shift your weight to the right. Turn your body to the right, and allow your left arm to naturally move downward, then upward to the middle line. Repeat this circling eight times.

■ Change direction of the circling. Begin with your weight on your left leg and your left arm extended, palm facing upward.

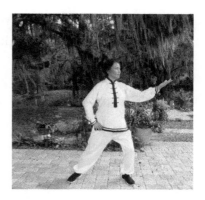

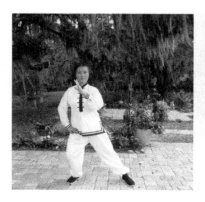 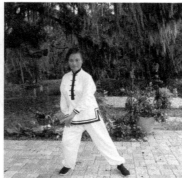

■ Shift your weight to the right, and allow your left arm and hand to naturally circle inward and downward.

- Shift your weight to the left, and allow your arm to move outward and upward.

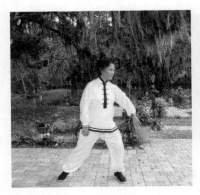 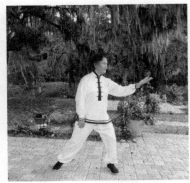

Your hand rotates naturally; no need to do anything special. Your arm needs to follow your body weight. "Body moves, arm follows"—I say this all the time when teaching. Do not intentionally move your arm; just follow the body. Circle eight times.

4. RIGHT HAND CIRCLES OUTWARD, THEN CIRCLES INWARD

You now change the arm and hand.

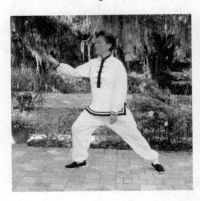 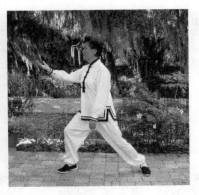

- Shift your weight to the right. Allow your right arm to naturally circle from the lower dan tian (lower abdomen) upward, then outward. Next shift your weight to the left, and allow your right arm to naturally sweep downward to the left and then upward. Do this eight times. You will finish with your weight and your right arm to your right.

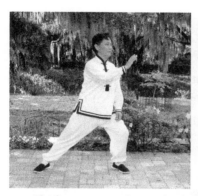
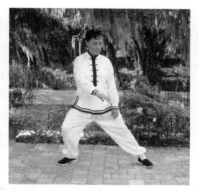

- Shift your weight to the left. Your right arm crosses to the left, in front of your chest, and sweeps down. Shift your weight back to the right. Your right arm circles back to the right, across your abdomen. Do this eight times.

Change the direction of the circling: shift your weight to the left, and then allow your right arm and hand to naturally circle inward and downward. When you shift your weight to the right, your arm moves outward and upward.

Your hand rotates naturally; no need to do anything special. Again, your arm needs to follow your body weight: "body moves, arm follows." Do not intentionally move your arm; just follow your body. Repeat this eight times.

5. BOTH HANDS CIRCLE OUTWARD, THEN INWARD

This is like the movement in the taiji form known as "wave hands like clouds" but involves movement from a stationary position, not walking.

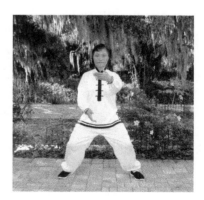

- Start in horse stance, and hold the left hand, palm facing inward, at chest level. The right hand is near the lower dan tian.

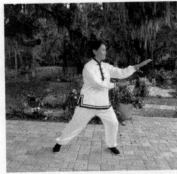

- The left arm circles outward as you turn and shift 70 percent of your weight to the left. At the same time, the right hand moves to the left.

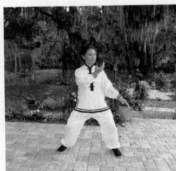 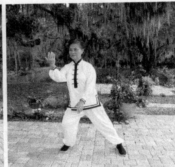 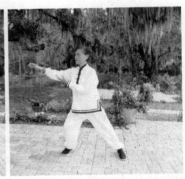

- Shift your weight and turn your waist to the right. The right hand circles outward to the right, and the left hand circles downward, then inward, and then to the right. As long as you maintain the circle, all you need to do is one arm at a time.

- Again, shift your weight and your arms to the left, and circle the arms. Continue to alternately shift from left to right. Make sure your arms are following the shifting of your weight.

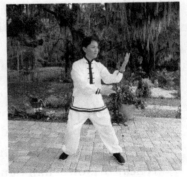

After eight repetitions, change the direction of the circles. As your weight shifts to the left, the right arm circles inward. As your shift your weight to the right, the left arm circles inward.

6. BOTH HANDS CIRCLE LEFT, THEN CIRCLE RIGHT

This exercise is not difficult.

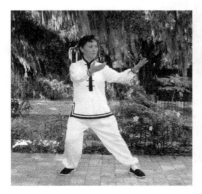 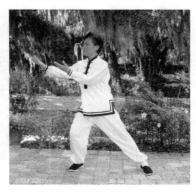

- With your weight shifted to your right, circle hands to the left at shoulder level. Imagine you are holding a big paintbrush with both hands apart and paint a large circle on the wall clockwise.

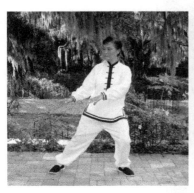 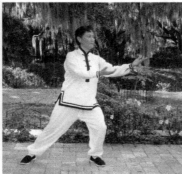

- The hands follow the body as the body shifts and turns back to the starting point.

7. LEFT SIDE 45-DEGREE CIRCLE ARM OUTWARD, THEN INWARD

This is similar to the third and fourth basic exercises above, but for this exercise, you step forward 45 degrees from the center.

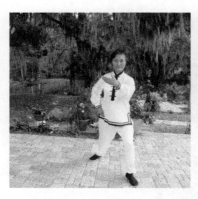 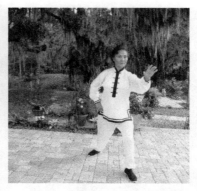

- Step forward 45 degrees from the center with your left foot, and circle your left arm outward. Follow your weight, shifting to the left foot.

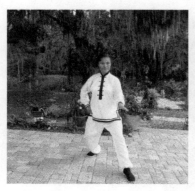 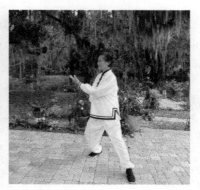

- Shift your weight to the right, circle your arm downward, and then circle inward to the middle line. Repeat this circle eight times.

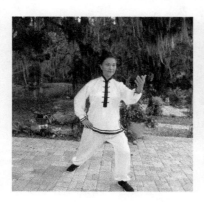 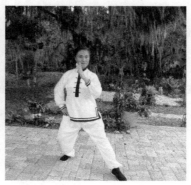

- Next reverse the circle. The left arm circles inward, then downward following the weight shifting to the right foot.

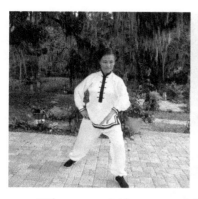 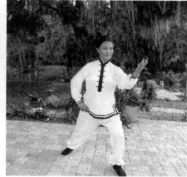

- When you shift your weight to the left foot, circle your arm outward, then upward. Repeat this circle eight times. Bring your left foot back next to your right foot.

8. RIGHT SIDE 45-DEGREE CIRCLE ARM OUTWARD, THEN INWARD

This is same as the above except step forward 45 degrees from center with your right foot.

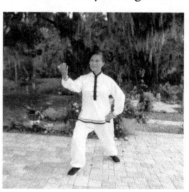

- Step forward with your right foot 45 degrees from center, and circle your right arm outward following your weight shifting to the right foot.

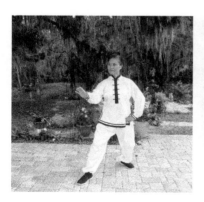 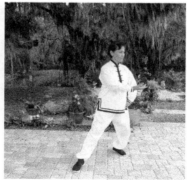

- Shift your weight to the left foot, and circle your arm downward. Then circle inward to the middle line. Repeat this eight times.

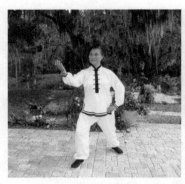 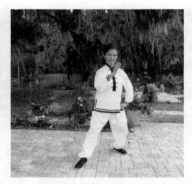

■ Reverse the circle. Your right arm circles inward, then downward following your weight shifting to the left foot.

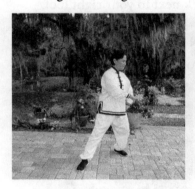 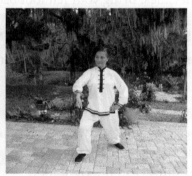

■ When you shift your weight to the right, circle your arm outward and upward. Repeat this circle eight times, then step back.

9. LEFT SIDE 45-DEGREE CIRCLE BOTH HANDS OUTWARD, THEN CIRCLE INWARD

This is similar to the fifth basic exercise (both hands circle outward, then inward), but you step forward 45 degrees with the left foot.

■ Step forward at a 45 degree angle with your left leg. The left arm circles outward as you turn and shift 70 percent of your weight to the left leg. At the same time, the right hand moves to the left.

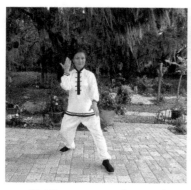 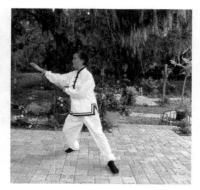

- Shift your weight, and turn your waist to the right. The right hand circles outward to the right, and the left hand circles downward, then inward, and then to the right.

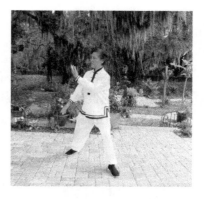

- Again, shift your weight to the left leg, and circle the arms. Continue alternately shifting from left to right. Make sure your arms are following the shifting of your weight.

After eight repetitions, change the direction of the circles.

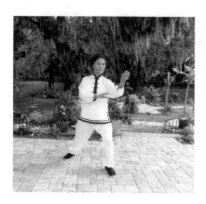

- Start with 70 percent of your weight on your left leg. Your left hand, palm facing inward, is at shoulder height, and your right hand, palm facing downward, is at chest level.

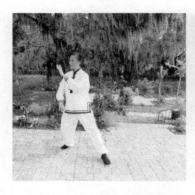 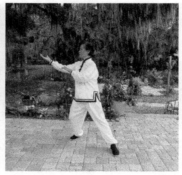

- Shift your weight to the right, and turn your waist to the right. As you shift, the left arm circles inward, then downward. Your right hand circles inward, then outward.

10. RIGHT SIDE 45-DEGREE CIRCLE BOTH HANDS OUTWARD, THEN CIRCLE INWARD

This is the same as the ninth basic exercise (left side 45-degree circle both hands outward, then circle inward), except you step forward with the right foot.

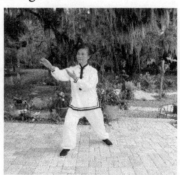

- Step forward at a 45 degree angle with your right leg. The right arm circles outward as you turn and shift 70 percent of your weight to the right leg. At the same time, the left hand moves to the right.

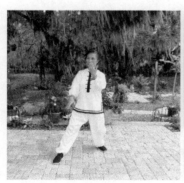 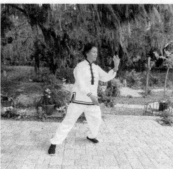 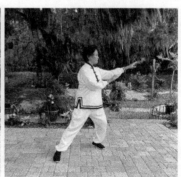

- Shift your weight to the left leg, and turn your waist to the left. The left hand circles outward to the left, and the right hand circles downward, then inward, and then to the left.

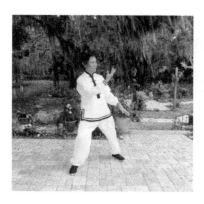

■ Again, shift your weight to the right foot, and circle the arms. Continue alternately shifting from left to right. Make sure your arms are following the shifting of your weight.

After eight repetitions, change the direction of the circles.

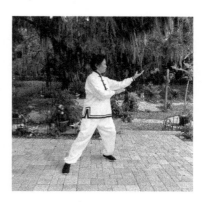

■ Start with 70 percent of your weight on your left leg. Your left hand, palm facing inward, is at shoulder height, and your right hand, palm facing downward, is at chest level.

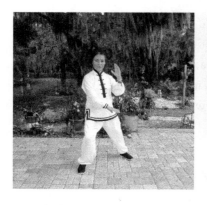 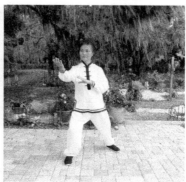

■ Shift your weight to the right, and turn your waist to the right. As you shift, the left arm circles inward, then downward. Your right hand circles inward, then outward.

11. BRUSH PUSH WITH RIGHT PALM

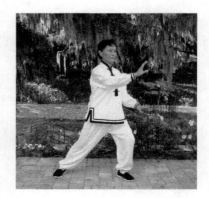

- Step forward with the left foot. Shift your weight to the right, the left arm circles inward, while the right arm circles downward and outward to shoulder level. Shift your weight to the left, the right hand pushes forward while the left arm naturally moves to the front of the left hip. Repeat this eight times. Step back.

12. BRUSH PUSH WITH LEFT PALM

Step forward with the right foot. Shift your weight to the left. The right arm circles inward, while the left arm circles downward and outward to shoulder level. Shift your weight to the right. The left hand pushes forward while the right arm naturally moves to the front of the right hip. Repeat this eight times. Step back.

13. HORSE STANCE PRACTICE

Horse stance practice is fundamental to every Chinese martial art practice. To do it correctly may take some time. It is good for your lower back and helps you to relax, be grounded, rooted, and more focused. It also helps to build core energy. The term *core energy* has different meanings in Eastern and Western thought. The Western approach focuses on building stronger abdominal muscles while the Eastern approach focuses on energy in the middle part of the body, the lower abdomen area, not necessarily on strong muscles. It is the energy part that I have a hard time explaining to people. People sometimes want to see it before they believe in it. They can see a "six-pack" of abdominal muscles, but they cannot see energy, what we call qi, or the body's powerhouse.

<u>Here is how you do it</u>

Step to the left so that your feet are a little wider than shoulder width apart. Relax your entire body from head to toe. Inhale, and raise your upper arms. The rest of the arms just go with the upper arms. Exhale, and sink the entire pelvis (sink your tailbone and your body will follow), bending your knees. At the same time, your elbows and arms are naturally following the sinking movement of the body. Your upper body is now vertical to the ground but relaxed. You will notice the relaxation of your arms as soon as you sink your elbows. You can place your arms in front of the body either forming a circle like you are hugging a big tree or just keeping your palms facing forward in front of your chest. In the position you are now in, you should feel very relaxed. Your body should feel rooted, grounded, centered, and strong like a big tree. Stay in this position for as long as you can. Beginners can stay in this position for one minute, then two minutes, gradually adding more time. If you do it correctly, five minutes should be no problem. Some people can do it for ten to thirty minutes.

Part 2: Taiji Walking (Cat Walk)

The importance of the "cat walk" is in its slow, smooth, well-controlled, and relaxed movements. If you don't relax, you will have a hard time controlling your walk. So just relax.

CAT WALK 1 (WALKING FORWARD)

With your feet a little more than shoulder width apart, relax your body and unlock your knees. Put weight onto your right foot. Step forward with your left foot (about 45 degrees off the centerline); the heel touches the floor first. Then shift your weight onto your left foot (60–70 percent). As you shift all your weight onto your left foot, slowly lift your right foot and move the right foot next to the left foot. In a continuous motion, move your right foot forward (about 45 degrees off centerline); the heel touches the floor first. Shift your weight onto the right foot and slowly lift your left foot and move your left foot next to your right foot.

CAT WALK 2 (WALKING FORWARD WITH WEIGHT SHIFTING, TURNING)

This walk is similar to cat walk 1 but has weight shifting in the middle of the walk. Relax your body, and unlock your knees. Put weight onto your right foot. Step forward with the left foot (about 45 degrees off centerline); the heel touches the floor first. Then shift your weight onto your left foot (60–70 percent). Shift weight back to the right foot (30–40 percent), and slightly turn your body to the left. Slowly shift weight onto your left foot again. At the same time, slowly lift your right foot, and move your right foot next to your left foot. In a continuous motion, move your right foot forward (about 45 degrees off centerline); the heel touches the floor first. Shift your weight onto your right foot (about 60–70 percent). Shift your weight back to the left (30–40 percent), and slightly turn your body to the right. Slowly shift your weight onto your right foot again. At the same time, slowly lift your left foot. Move your left foot next to your right foot.

CAT WALK 3 (WALKING BACKWARD)

This is backward walking. Unlock your knees, and put weight on your right foot. Slowly step back with the left foot (about 45 degrees off centerline); the toe touches the floor first. Place your heel down at a natural angle. Shift your weight onto your left foot. At the same time, adjust the right foot to put the body into a comfortable and natural stance.

Lift your right foot. Slowly step back with your right foot (about 45 degrees off centerline); the toe touches the floor first. Place your heel down at a natural angle. Shift your weight onto your right foot. At the same time, adjust your left foot to put the body into a comfortable and natural stance.

CAT WALK 4 (WALKING SIDEWAYS)

Unlock your knees, and shift your weight onto your right foot. Slowly step to your left. Your toes touch the floor first. It is not necessary to take a big step. It should be a comfortable step. Slowly shift your weight onto your left foot. At the same time, lift your right foot. Bring the right foot next to the left foot about one fist away, toe down first. Then shift your weight onto your right foot, and step left again, completing the sequence again. Step four or five times to the left, then step four or five times to the right.

Part 3: Taiji Qigong (Exercise Sequence)

This is a short qigong form with taiji movements in stationary practice. Everyone seems to love this short taiji qigong practice.

1. PREPARATION

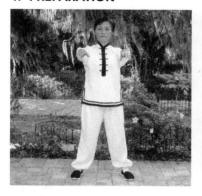 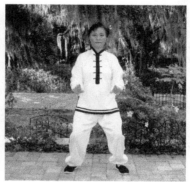

- Step to the left so your feet are shoulder width apart or a little wider. Inhale, and raise your arms to shoulder height. Then exhale, and sink your body and elbows, forming a horse stance.

2. WARDOFF

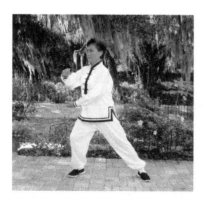

- Shift your weight to the right, and turn to the right. The left hand tucks under the right arm. It feels like you are holding a ball on your right side.

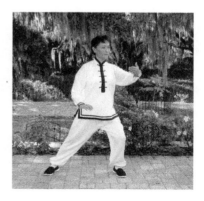

- Shift your weight to the left, and move your left hand out to the left 45 degrees. The right hand gently presses down next to hip.

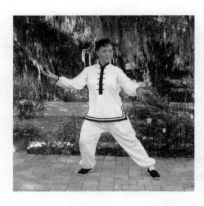

- Shift your weight to the right. The arms naturally open.

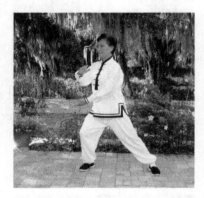

- Then place your left hand under the right elbow, like you are holding a ball on your right side.

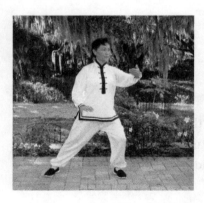

- Shift your weight onto your left leg, and move your left hand out to the left 45 degrees. The right hand gently presses down next to the hip.

    Repeat this movement four times.

3. BRUSH PUSH

- Start from the end of wardoff.

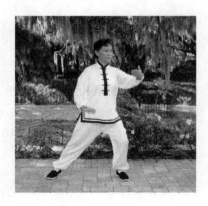

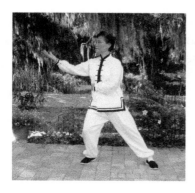

■ Shift your weight to the right. The left arm circles inward, while the right arm circles outward to shoulder level.

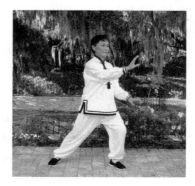

■ Shift your weight to the left. The right hand pushes to the left 45 degrees as you are shifting your weight to the left. The left hand moves naturally to the front of the left hip.

Shift your weight to the right as the left hand pushes forward and the right arm naturally moves to the front of the right hip. Do this sequence eight times.

4. WIND BLOWS THE WILLOW TREE

This is a nice and easy movement. It is perfect for practicing shifting and turning.

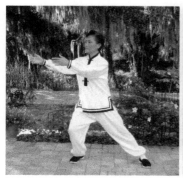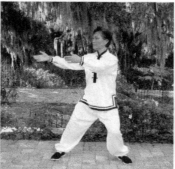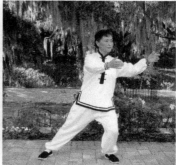

■ Shift your weight, and turn your waist from the right to the left. Move your arms following your body weight shifting and turning. When you shift your weight to the left, the arms follow from right to left.

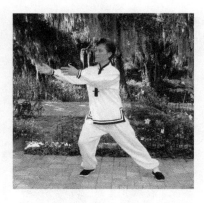

■ When you shift your weight and turn your waist to the right, move both arms to the right.

    Do this sequence eight times.

5. WAVE HANDS

■ Place your hands in front of the body, with the left hand in front of your chest and the right hand in front of your lower abdomen.

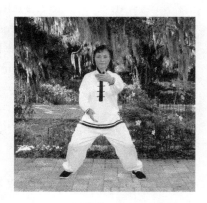

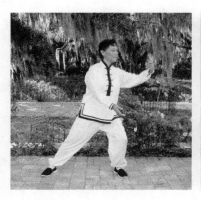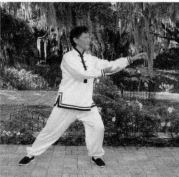

■ Shift your weight to the left, turning your waist to the left as well. At the same time, the left hand circles outward, and the right hand moves to the left.

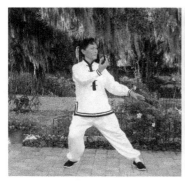 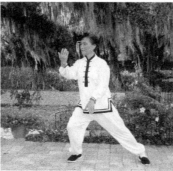 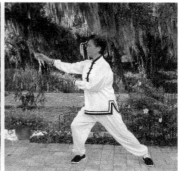

- Shift your weight, and turn your waist to the right. The right hand circles outward and then to the right. The left hand circles downward, then to the right. Do this sequence eight times.

6. BLOCK, LEAD, PRESS, AND PUSH

This is a set of continuous movements that allow you to feel the flow of the energy. You will become peaceful and relaxed.

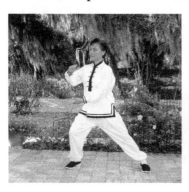

- As you shift your weight to the right, the left hand tucks under your right arm. It feels like you are holding a ball on your right side.

- Shift your weight to the left and move the left hand out to the left 45 degrees. The right hand gently presses down next to hip.

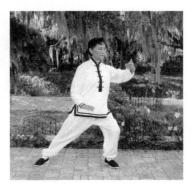

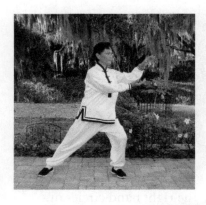

- The right hand comes up to meet the left hand like holding a smaller ball.

- Shift your weight to the right. As your waist turns, move your arms and hands downward, then upward to the right.

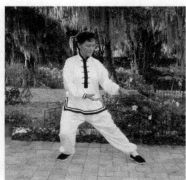

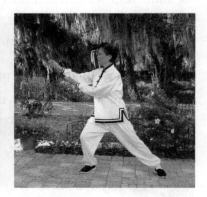

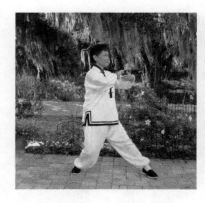

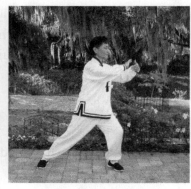

- Then continue the motion. Turn your body to the left, and shift your weight to the left leg. Move your arms and hands to the left.

- Shift your weight from the left leg to the right leg. Relax both hands and arms. You are still facing to the left.

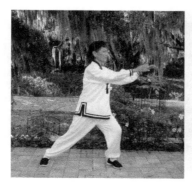 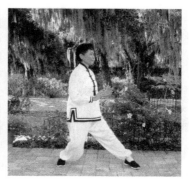

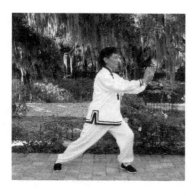

- Shift your weight back to your left leg, and push both palms forward in front of the body.

7. CIRCLE ARMS, MOVE QI THROUGH THE BODY (ENDING)

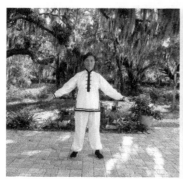 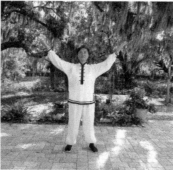 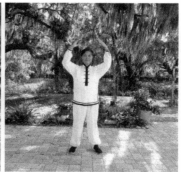

- Feet are shoulder width apart. Inhale, and raise your arms along the sides of your body until they are above your head.

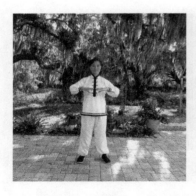 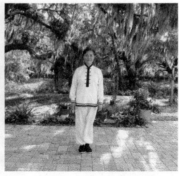

■ Exhale, and move arms and hands down in front of the body. Do this sequence three times.

Part 4: Taiji Thirteen Movements

The taiji thirteen movements are the most important in the taiji form. Learning these movements helps you to learn the taiji form much more easily, especially after practicing taiji basics or taiji qigong. Not only do you get taiji benefits from these movements, but they are also very enjoyable.

1. WUJI POSITION

Wu means "nothing"; ji means "one extreme." Wuji here means no left, no right, no up or down—completely neutral.

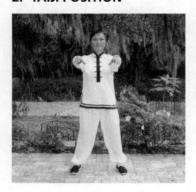

■ With feet should width apart, relax your body and mind. Your arms are naturally on the sides of the body with no tension. Breathe deeply and slowly.

2. TAIJI POSITION

■ Raise your arms to shoulder level as you breathe in.

- Sink the tailbone and elbows as you breathe out. You are now in horse stance. Your hands are in front of your hips. Your mind is focused on your body and your breath. You should feel very relaxed and comfortable.

    Do this sequence four to eight times.

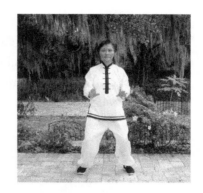

3. SEPARATE HANDS (WARDOFF)

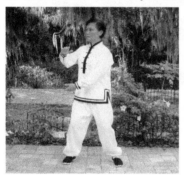

- Shift your weight onto the right foot. The left hand tucks under the right arm like you are holding a ball on your right side. Your right hand is positioned as if resting on the top of the ball.

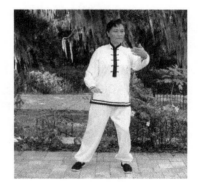

- The left foot steps forward slightly off center. Shift 70 percent of your weight onto your left leg. At the same time, your left hand moves out to the front of the body at chin level. The right hand gently moves down to the right hip level.

Now perform the same movement on the other side.

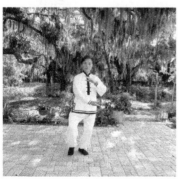

- Step back with the left foot, and bring the right hand under the left like you are holding a ball on your left side.

- The right foot steps forward slightly off center. Shift 70 percent of your weight onto the right leg. At the same time, your right hand moves out to the front of the body at chin level. The left hand gently moves down to the left hip level.

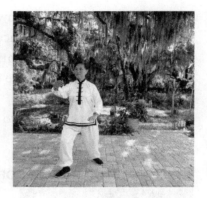

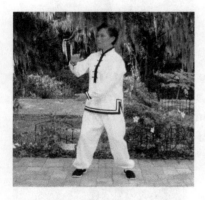

- Step back with the right foot, and hold the ball on the right side.

   Do this sequence eight times.

4. ROLL BACK ARM

- Start in horse stance.

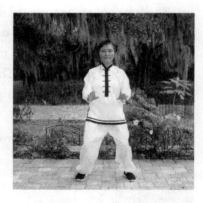

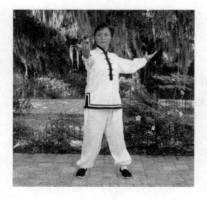

- Inhale, and turn your body to the left. At the same time, move your right arm to the front of the body and the left arm back to the body 45 degrees off centerline, palms at shoulder level. Both palms are facing up.

- Exhale, and bring the left hand close to your left ear.

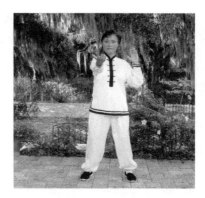

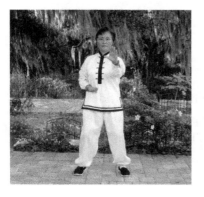

- Then push your left hand forward, palm out. At the same time, move your right arm back to waist level.

- Inhale, and let your right arm and hand naturally circle back outward until both hands are at shoulder level, with both palms facing up and the elbows slightly bent. The body is naturally turning to the right.

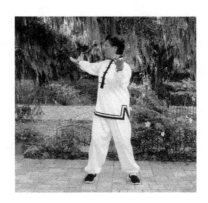

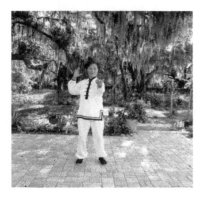

- Exhale, and bring your right hand close to your right ear.

- Then push your right hand forward. At the same time, move your left arm back to waist level.

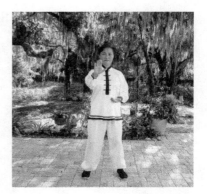

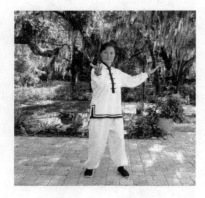

- Inhale, and let the left arm and hand naturally circle back until the palm is at shoulder level, elbows slightly bent. Both palms are now facing up. The body is naturally turning to the right.

Do this movement to the right and the left eight times.

5. WAVE HANDS

We have discussed this earlier, in the section on taiji qigong, but here again, we practice this movement because it is an important one.

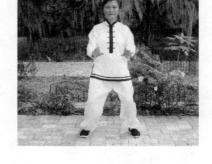

- Start in horse stance.

Place your left hand in front of your chest and your right hand in front of your lower abdomen.

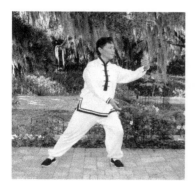

- Shift your weight, and turn your waist to the left. Your arms naturally follow the body in a circular

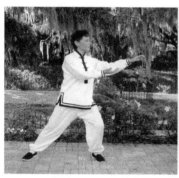 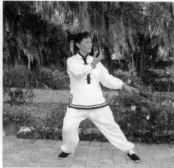 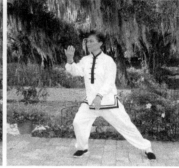

- When your body is shifting and turning from the left to the right, the left arm circles outward, then downward, and the right arm circles inward, then upward.

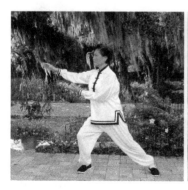 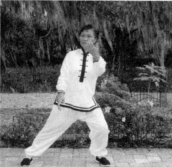 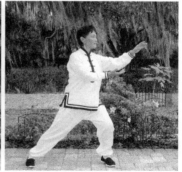

- When your body is shifting and turning from the right to the left, the right arm circles outward, then downward, and the left arm circles inward, then upward.

6. BRUSH PUSH (VARIATION)

Brush push is similar to the eleventh and twelfth exercises in the section "Taiji Basics" above but a little different. (You also saw brush push in the section on taiji qigong, although this version is slightly different.) It is an important movement.

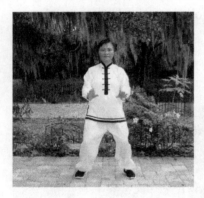

- Start in horse stance.

- Shift your weight to the right. The left arm circles inward, while the right arm circles outward to shoulder level. Step forward (45 degrees off centerline) with the left foot, heel down. As you put weight onto your left foot, your right hand pushes forward, and your left hand naturally moves to the left hip level.

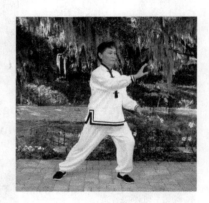

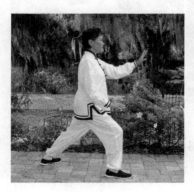

- Step back with the left foot, then put weight on it. Place both arms on the left side at shoulder level, step forward with the right foot (45 degrees off centerline). As you shift weight onto your right foot, your left hand pushes forward, and your right hand naturally moves to the right hip level.

7. PLAY GUITAR

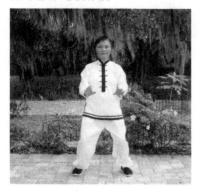

- Start in horse stance.

- Shift your weight onto your right leg, and extend your left leg, heel on the ground. Inhale slightly, and open your arms to the side. Exhale, and move the arms close to the centerline with the left hand at neck level, elbow slightly bent, and the right hand in front of the middle dan tian (middle abdomen) under the left elbow. The palms face toward the center.

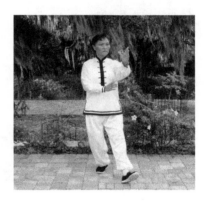

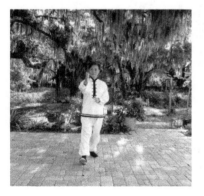

- Relax the arms and hands, and step back with your left foot. Putting your weight on your left foot, inhale and slightly open your arms to the side. Exhale, and move the arms close to the centerline with the right hand at neck level with elbow slightly bent and the left hand in front of the middle dan tian (middle abdomen) under the right elbow. The palms face toward the center.

Do this movement eight times.

8. DOUBLE PUNCH AT EAR LEVEL

- Start in horse stance.

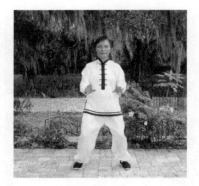

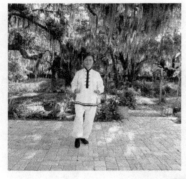

- Put your weight on your left foot. Put both hands on your waist making a soft fist.

- Step forward with your right foot as you shift weight to your right foot. Your fists punch forward to ear level.

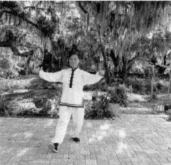

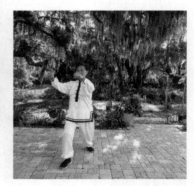

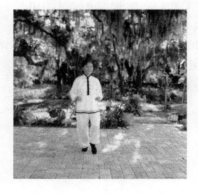

- Bring your right foot back next to your left foot. Put weight on your right foot. At the same time, bring your fists back to your waist.

- Step forward with your left foot. As you shift your weight to your left foot, your fists punch forward to ear level.

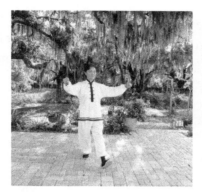 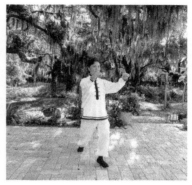

Bring your left foot back next to your right foot, returning to horse stance. At the same time, bring your fists back to your waist.

Do this movement eight times.

9. SINGLE LEG STANDING

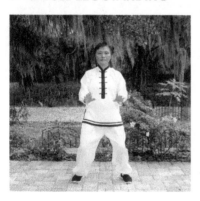

- Start in horse stance.

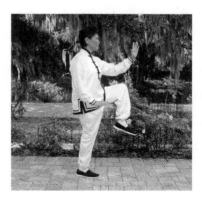

- Lift your left leg to hip level while lifting your left arm in front of your body. Sink the elbow. The palm faces forward, and your fingers are at eye level. Your right hand is next to your right hip.

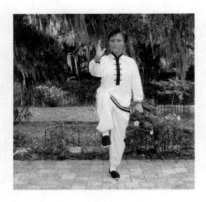

- Gently step down. Your left palm moves next to your left hip. Lift your right leg to hip level, while lifting your right arm in front of your body. Sink your elbow. Your palm faces forward, and your fingers are at eye level. Your left hand is next to your left hip.

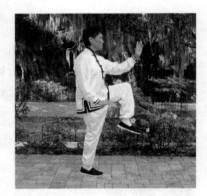

- Gently step down. Your right palm moves next to your right hip.

    Repeat this movement four to eight times.

10. GRASP THE BIRD'S TAIL

This very important sequence needs to be carefully learned and practiced. You can feel the moving qi in this group of taiji movements. Practice slowly and mindfully. Coordinating with your breath is key.

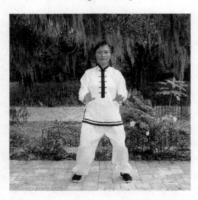

- Start in horse stance.

■ Put weight on your right foot, holding an imaginary ball on your right side with the left hand under the right arm, right hand on top. Step out with your left foot.

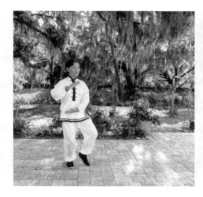 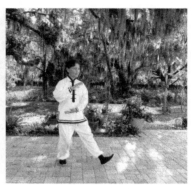

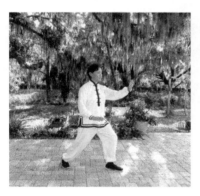

■ Shifting your weight onto your left foot, move your left hand to chin level, elbow slightly bent, and move the right hand next to the right hip.

■ Move your right hand across your body under the left palm, palms facing each other.

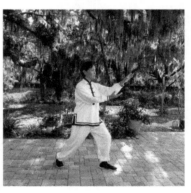

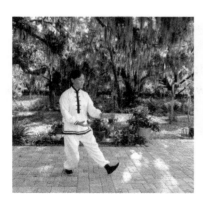 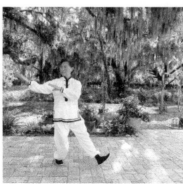

■ Shifting your weight right, move both arms right until your hands are at shoulder level.

- Shifting your weight left, move both hands left, palms facing each other, like holding a small ball at chest level. You are facing left.

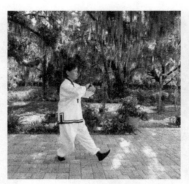 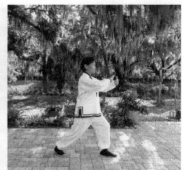

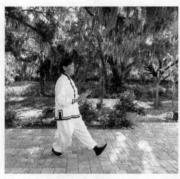 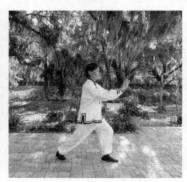

- Shift your weight back to your right foot (sit back). Bring both hands to the lower dan tian (lower abdomen). Shift your weight left, and push palms forward (facing left) with elbows slightly bent.

    Do this movement to the right.

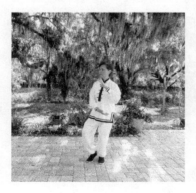

- Put weight on your left foot, holding an imaginary ball on your left side with the right hand under the left arm, left hand on top. Step out with your right foot.

■ Shifting your weight right, move your right hand to chin level, elbow slightly bent, and move the left hand next to the left hip.

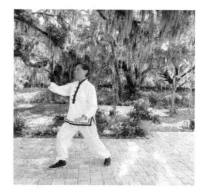

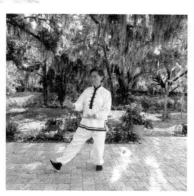

■ Move your left hand across your body under the right palm, palms facing each other.

■ Shifting your weight left, move both arms left until your hands are at shoulder level.

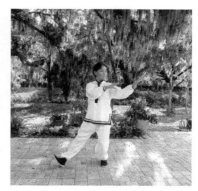

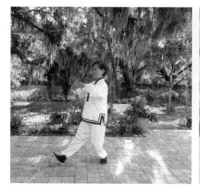

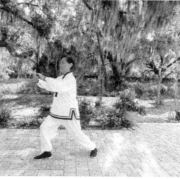

■ Shifting your weight right, move both hands right, palms facing each other, like holding a small ball at chest level. You are facing right.

- Shifting your weight back to your left foot (sit back), bring both hands to the lower dan tian (lower abdomen).

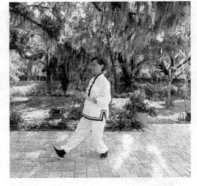

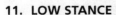

- Shift your weight right, and push your palms forward (facing right) with elbows slightly bent. Repeat this movement.

11. LOW STANCE

- Start in horse stance.

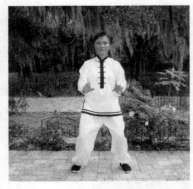

- Put weight on your right leg, and place both arms to the right side. The fingers of the right hand are all together, pointing downward.

- Step far to the left with the left foot. Bend your right leg, and lower your body into a deep stance while your left hand sweeps toward your left foot, and your right arm remains in position, following the movement naturally.

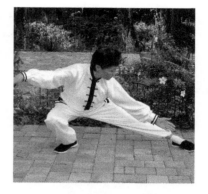

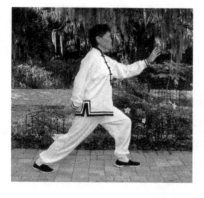

- Shift your weight to the left foot. As you shift, move your left hand downward, then upward.

- In continuous motion, lift your right leg, pressing your left palm down next to your hip. The right hand moves downward, then upward until it is in front of the body with elbow pointing downward and fingers at eye level pointing up. At the same time, lift the right leg. The left hand gently presses down next to the left hip.

  Continue to the other side.

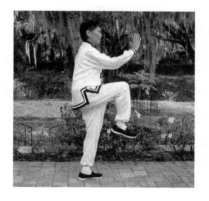

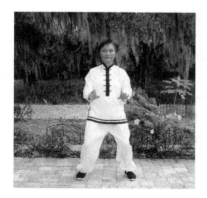

- Start again in horse stance.

- Put weight on your left leg, and place both arms to the left side. The fingers of the left hand are all together, pointing downward.

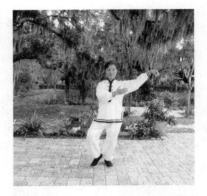

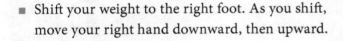

- Step far to the right with the right foot. Bend your left leg, and lower your body into a deep stance while your right hand sweeps toward your right foot, and your left arm remains in position, simply following the movement naturally.

- Shift your weight to the right foot. As you shift, move your right hand downward, then upward.

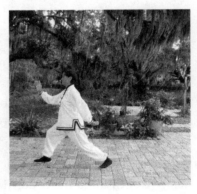

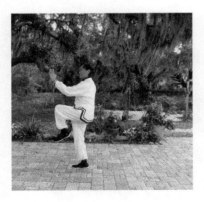

- In continuous motion, lift your left leg, pressing your right palm down next to your hip. The left hand moves downward, then upward until it is in front of the body with elbow pointing downward and fingers at eye level pointing up. At the same time, lift the left leg. The right hand gently presses down next to the right hip.
  Do this movement four times.

12. KICKING

- Start in horse stance.

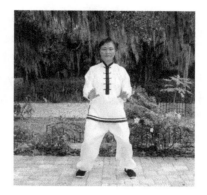

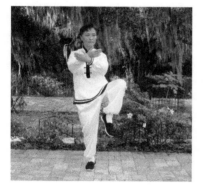

- Put all your weight on the right leg. Lift the left leg, and at the same time, move your arms to the front of your body with wrists crossed.

- Continue to lift the left leg, then kick forward. At the same time, open the arms to your sides. The left arm is over the left leg, and the right arm is on the right side of the body.

  Continue to the other side.

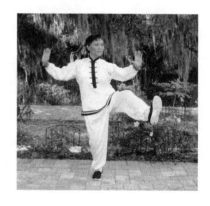

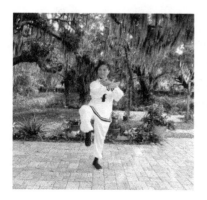

- Step down with the left foot, and put all your weight on your left leg. Lift the left leg, and at the same time, move your arms to the front of your body with wrists crossed.

■ Continue to lift the right leg, then kick forward. At the same time, open the arms to the sides. The right arm is over the right leg, and the left arm is on the left side of the body.

Do this movement four to eight times.

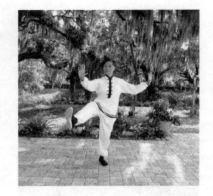

13. FAIR LADY MOVES THE SHUTTLE

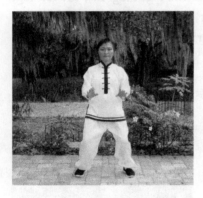

■ Start in horse stance.

■ Put your weight on the left leg. The right hand moves under the left arm, like holding a ball on your left side.

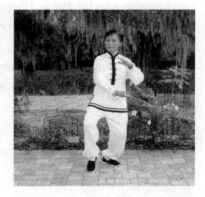

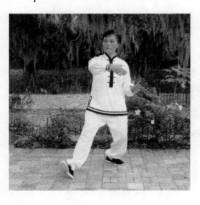

■ Step forward 45 degrees with your right foot. At the same time, change the dimension of your hands, with the left hand next to your middle waist.

- As you shift your weight to your right foot, push the left hand forward slightly off middle line to the right. At the same time, move the right arm up to the right slightly above the right temple, about six inches away.

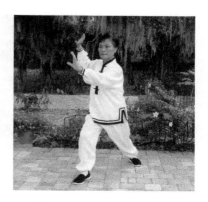

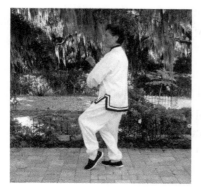

- Continue to the other side. Shift weight back, bringing the right foot back next to the left foot. Put weight on the right leg, with the left hand under the right arm like holding a ball on your right side.

- Step forward 45 degrees with the left foot. As you shift weight to the left foot, push the right arm forward slightly to the left. At the same time, move the left arm up to the left slightly above the left temple, about six inches away. Shift weight back, bringing the left foot back next to the right foot. Do this movement four times.

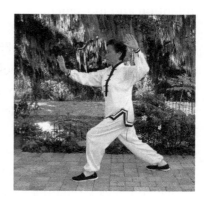

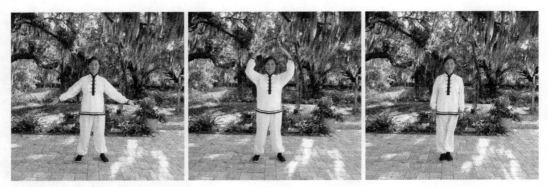

- To end, take a slow, deep breath, and raise your arms up from the side of your body. Exhale, and lower your arms down in front of your body.

QI PRACTICE (FOUNDATION PRACTICE)

Qi practice is used in every taiji movement, especially during foundation practice. Some people already know some qigong and use their qigong form to do a qi practice. During qi practice, you must remove any thoughts, focus on your awareness of every part of the body, and also relax every part of the body. If you move the body, keep your focus on the center of the body, move slowly, and incorporate your breath with your intention and movement.

FORM PRACTICE (MOVING QI PRACTICE)

This is what most people do. Following this guideline will allow you to learn and practice the form well. It makes your learning easier and your practice effective and enjoyable. It does not matter what form you do or learn. It can be any form of taiji.

STRETCHING

Stretching should be done before and after practice. When stretching after taiji, mostly do leg and back stretching because these parts of the body are used most in taiji practice. You can do whole-body stretching if you wish.

COOLDOWN AND ENDING

Some people use qi practice to cool down, and some people use meditation to cool down. You can do both; it is totally up to you. When you finish your taiji practice, you can take a slow deep breath to allow the qi to move through the whole body.

Twenty-Four-Step Yang-Style Taijiquan Form

People tell me it is not easy to learn taiji from a book, TV, or YouTube. In some ways it is true, but you can still learn taiji from a book and other ways. If the book has a structured teaching system, you can learn with minimum difficulty. Eventually, however, you will need a good teacher who can guide you to deeper learning and practicing.

If you are an instructor, this book will help you to provide the structured teaching students need. This helps them feel good about their learning. They have better focus, more energy, more calmness, a clearer mind, better circulation, and better movement. On the other hand, you will get more joy from teaching; not only will you feel good, but you will also see your students do well with their form and have a positive attitude.

Learning taiji, you must understand the real relaxation practice: effortlessly produce results. This is Dao, the wisdom that helps in every area of life. The interesting thing is that the harder you try, the worse you feel. It is like everything else: if you try too hard, the results are never what you expect. Learning taiji starts with relaxation, which applies to every single movement. Go with the flow, and then the energy will flow. You will learn to move the body without raising muscle tension. Raise only your mind's intention. Then everything will become easy.

Twenty-four step taiji is the most popular form. Almost everyone in China who has learned taiji knows this form. Many people who practice taiji in other countries know this form too. This is a good thing because you can easily join a taiji group when you see people practice this form either in China or elsewhere. If you are in China, you will see people in the morning practice taiji on the street or in a park. Even in the United States, you will see more people who know this form than any other form.

The names of the steps have many translations. You may see the same movement but with a different name. No matter the translation, the movement is the same. In the next chapter, "Ten-Week Learning Guidelines," we will discuss the detailed movements of the twenty-four-step Yang-style form.

Names of the Steps:

1. Taiji preparation
2. Parting the wild horse's mane (wardoff)
3. White crane spreads its wings
4. Brush knee
5. Play the guitar
6. Step back, roll back the arms (repulse monkey)
7. Grasp the bird's tail, on the left
8. Grasp the bird's tail, on the right
9. Single whip
10. Wave hands like clouds
11. Single whip
12. Gauge the height of the horse (high pat on horse)
13. Right kick
14. Strike the ear with fist
15. Turn body and left kick
16. Left low stance, stand on left leg (snake creeping down, golden pheasant standing on left leg)
17. Right low stance, stand on right leg (snake creeping down, golden pheasant standing on right leg)
18. Move the shuttle, left then right (fair lady moves the shuttle)
19. Pick needle from the sea
20. Send a flash through the arms
21. Turn body, deflect, block, and punch

22. Pull back, then push

23. Cross hands

24. Taiji ending, closing position

CHAPTER 5

Ten-Week Learning Guidelines

THESE TEN-WEEK learning guidelines are to make it easier for you to start your learning journey. And you don't have to just do ten weeks. You can make it twenty or thirty weeks if you wish. For instance, you can do the week-one lesson over two or three weeks. If you do want to get it down in ten weeks, you must learn and practice every single day, sixty minutes each time at least.

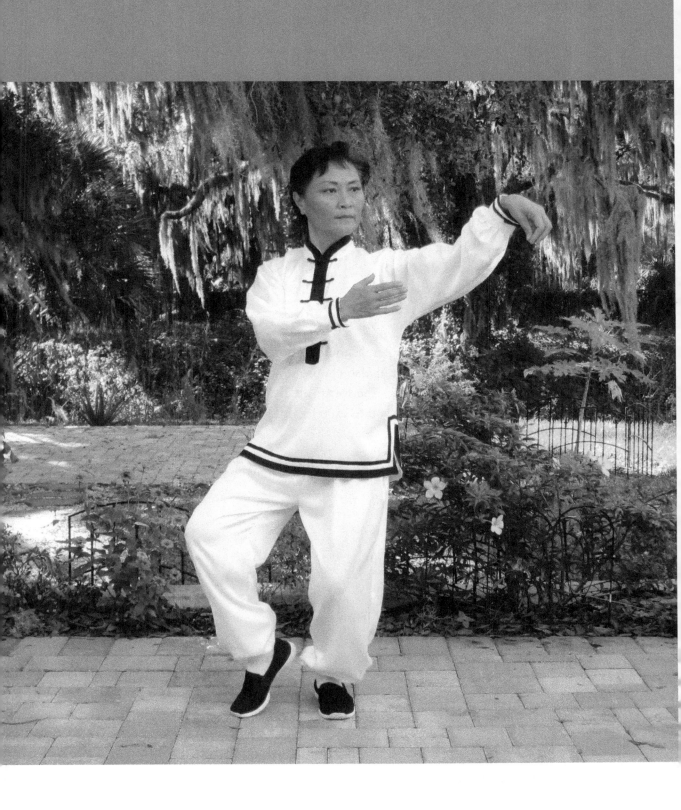

Week 1

1. Learn the warm-up exercises.

2. Practice the taiji stances.

3. Practice taiji walking (cat walk): forward and backward, then to the left and right. See below.

4. Practice taiji basics from chapter 4.

1. WARM-UP EXERCISES

The warm-up exercises from chapter 4 should be done every time you practice taiji. As we noted in that section, you could also choose to walk or jog fifteen to twenty minutes and do some light stretching. The warm-up exercises from chapter 4 are helpful when the weather doesn't permit you to exercise outdoors.

2. TAIJI STANCES

In this taiji form, there are six stances. Other forms may involve different stances.

HORSE STANCE

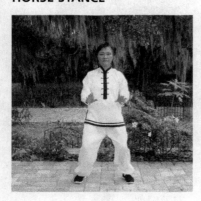

■ Horse stance.

The first taiji stance is horse stance. As we discussed in chapter 4, horse stance has many benefits and is one of the most important stances among all Chinese martial arts, including taiji. It has to be done correctly; otherwise, you may do more harm than good. The instructions for horse stance appeared in chapter 4, but I repeat them here for convenience's sake, with the addition of a short energy circulation exercise.

1. Step to the left so that your feet are a little wider than shoulder width. Relax your entire body from head to toe.

2. Inhale, and raise your upper arms. The rest of the arms just go with the upper arms. Exhale, and sink the entire pelvis (sink your tailbone and your body will follow), bending your knees. At the same time, your elbows and arms are naturally following the sinking movement of the body. Your upper body is now vertical to the ground but relaxed. You will notice the relaxation of your arms as soon as you sink your elbows.

3. You can place your arms in front of the body either forming a circle like you are hugging a big tree or just keeping your palms facing forward in front of the chest. In the position you are now in, you should feel very relaxed. Your body should feel rooted, grounded, centered, and strong like a big tree.

4. Stay in this position for as long as you can. Beginners can stay in this position for one minute, then two minutes, gradually adding more time. If you do it correctly, five minutes should be no problem. Some people can do it for ten to thirty minutes.

5. Breathe slowly and deeply. With each inhalation, visualize drawing energy from the earth into your body. With each exhalation, visualize moving energy back into the earth. In this way, form a circulation of energy between you and the earth.

You do not need to bend your knees very low unless you are a younger person and enjoy the challenge. Find your own comfort level.

WEEK 1

LUNGE STANCE (BOW STANCE)

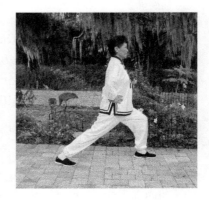

- Begin with your body upright and your feet one fist-width apart. Turn your right foot slightly to the right, and put weight on the right foot. Your left foot steps forward slightly off center. Bend your left knee, and put 70 percent of your weight on your left foot; the lower part of your left leg is vertical to the ground. Your right foot is somewhat straight and bears only 30 percent of the weight. Your body is still upright. After staying in this position for several breaths, bring the left foot back next to the right foot. Now perform the same movement but with your opposite leg.

SIDE LUNGE

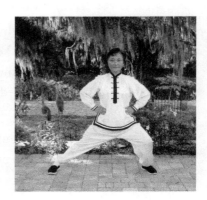

- Slowly step left so that your feet are shoulder width apart. When you exhale, put 70 percent of the weight on your left leg and 30 percent on your right. Your body is upright, the lower back relaxed. After several breaths, shift your weight to the right leg 70 percent, left leg 30 percent. Stay in this position for several breaths. Repeat several times.

EMPTY STANCE

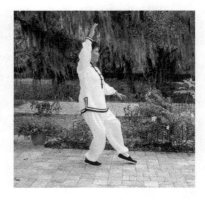

- Empty stance can sometimes confuse people. Empty means no body weight. Put 100 percent of your weight on your right leg, and relax your lower back. Slowly move your left toe forward to touch the floor but slightly off center. Your left toe bears no weight; it is just touching the floor, or bears just 5 percent of the weight if you have to. Hold this position for several breaths. Do the same thing with your right foot.

SIT-BACK STANCE

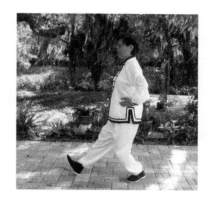

- Start with the left lunge (bow stance). Seventy percent of your weight is on your left leg. Shift your weight back to the right leg by bending the right knee and moving the hip back toward the right leg. Put 70 percent of your weight on the right leg. Hold for one to two breaths, then shift your weight forward onto the left foot, forming a lunge stance. Then shift your weight back, and hold for two breaths. Repeat this several times.

Change your stance to a right-lunge stance. Shift your weight back onto your left leg by bending your left knee and moving your hip back onto the left leg. Put 70 percent of the weight on the left leg. Hold for one to two breaths, then shift your weight forward onto the right foot, forming a lunge stance. Shift your weight back, and hold for two breaths. Repeat this several times.

LIFTING LEG

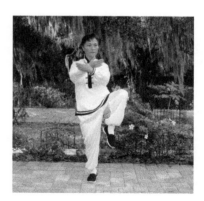

- Put weight on the right leg. Slowly lift the left leg until the knee is at hip level. Your foot is relaxed. Hold this position for several breaths. Do the same thing with the other leg. Repeat this several times.

3. TAIJI WALKING

In chapter 4 we noted that we also call taiji walk the cat walk and that there are four types of cat walk in taiji practice. All of the taiji walks (cat walks) can help you to improve your balance and build strong and rooted qi. See the section on taiji basics in chapter 4 for detailed explanations of how to perform the cat walks.

4. LEARNING TAIJI BASICS

We have discussed before that taiji basics are part of the building blocks. See "Taiji Basics" in chapter 4.

Week 2

1. Practice the warm-up exercises.

2. Practice the taiji stances.

3. Practice taiji walking (cat walk): forward and backward, then to the left and to the right. See week 1 practice.

4. Practice taiji basics from chapter 4, skipping taiji walking (cat walk) because you already performed it.

5. Learn taiji thirteen movements from chapter 4.

Week 3

1. Practice the warm-up exercises.
2. Practice taiji walking (cat walk): forward and backward, then to the left and to the right.
3. Practice taiji qigong from chapter 4.
4. Practice taiji thirteen movements. From chapter 4.
5. Learn movements 1–3 of the form:
    1. Taiji preparation
    2. Parting the wild horse's mane (wardoff)
    3. White crane spreads its wings

1. TAIJI PREPARATION

You will recall much of the below description of taiji position from chapter 4, in the section "Taiji Thirteen Movements." We begin from a different initial position, but everything else is the same.

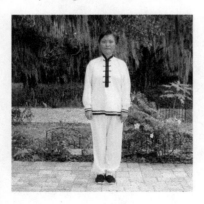

■ Begin in a neutral and relaxed upright position, feet together, arms relaxed, and head held upright with the chin slightly tucked down.

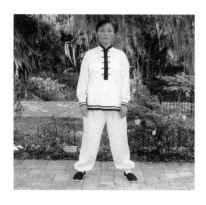

- Slowly step to the left while remaining relaxed. You are now in wuji position, which means completely neutral.

- Raise arms in front of the body until they reach shoulder level.

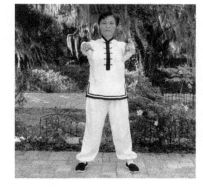

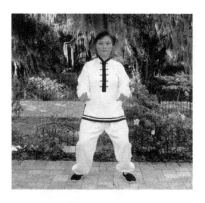

- Sink your tailbone and hips. Relax the lower back. You may need to tuck your buttocks to remove the curve of the lower back. At the same time, sink your elbows. The rest of your arm will just follow. You are now in taiji position.

2. PARTING THE WILD HORSE'S MANE (WARDOFF)

- Put your weight on your right leg. The left hand moves under the right arm like you are holding a ball on the right side. The right arm is lifted on the right side with the elbow bent just a little below shoulder level.

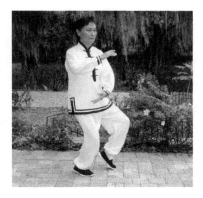

- The left foot steps to the left, heel first. Your body faces left.

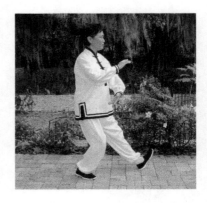

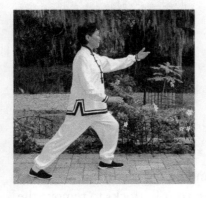

- Slowly shift your weight onto your left leg. Move your left hand out in front of the body to neck level, following the weight shifting. The right hand moves gently downward until it is next to the right hip.

- Shift your weight back to the right leg. Slightly turn your body to the left. At the same time, both arms naturally follow.

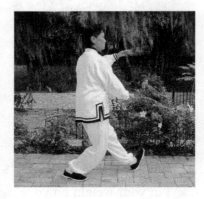

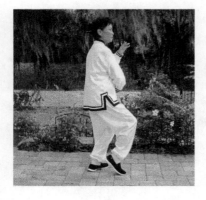

- Slowly bring your right foot next to the left foot. Your arms form the position like you are holding a ball on the left side.

- Then the right foot slowly steps forward, off the centerline, heel first (you are still facing left). Slowly shift your weight onto the right leg.

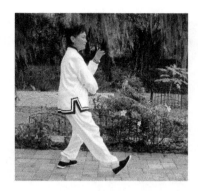

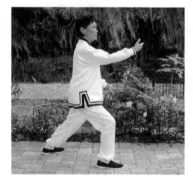

- Move your right hand out in front of the body until it reaches neck level. The movement follows the weight shifting. The left hand gently moves downward next to the left hip.

- Continue to the other side. Shift your weight back to the left leg. Slightly turn the body to the right. At the same time, both arms naturally follow.

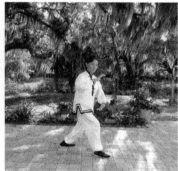

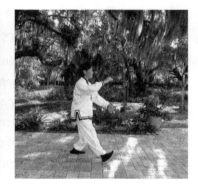

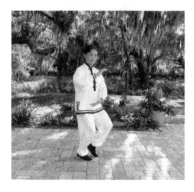

- Slowly bring the left foot next to the right foot (for the beginner, you can slide the foot on the floor). Your arms form a position like you are holding a ball on the right side.

- The left foot slowly steps forward, off the center-line, heel first. You will still be facing left.

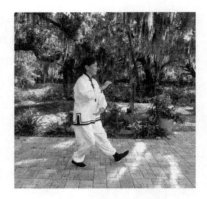

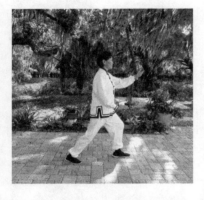

- Slowly shift your weight onto the left leg. Move the left hand out in front of the body until it is at neck level. The movements follow the weight shifting. The right hand gently moves downward to the level of the right hip.

3. WHITE CRANE SPREADS ITS WINGS

- Start from end of parting the wild horse's mane. Your weight is on the left leg. Continue to put weight on it. Bring the right foot halfway closer to the left foot. At the same time, your hands and arms are naturally placed in front of the body. It feels like you are holding a big ball in front of the body.

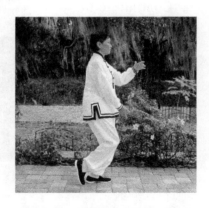

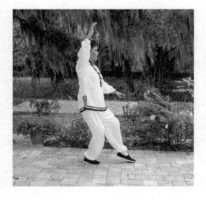

- As you step down the right foot and put weight on it, you raise your right arm up to the right, and move the left arm to the left side of the left hip. The left toe touches the floor. You are now in empty stance (see week one).

You have now completed the first three movements. You can repeat the three taiji movements as many times as you wish until you feel very relaxed and calm, with no tension in the body. Practice them until you can do these movements easily. You will need to make sure to do them slowly, mindfully, and while completely relaxed. Practice these every day for a whole week before moving on to next week's practice.

WEEK 3

Week 4

1. Practice the warm-up exercises.

2. Practice taiji basics.

3. Practice taiji qigong.

4. Practice taiji thirteen movements.

5. Learn movements 4–6 of the form:
   4. Brush knee
   5. Play the guitar
   6. Step back, roll back the arms (repulse the monkey)

6. Perform the taiji movements from 1 to 6 two times.

4. BRUSH KNEE

- Start from the end of white crane spreads its wings.

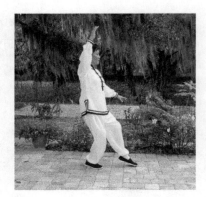

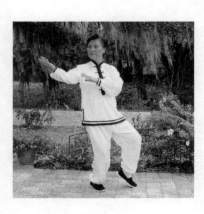

- Slightly turn your body to the right as you move the right arm down to the right slightly behind your body to shoulder level. The left arm circles inward to chest level.

- The left foot steps forward, heel first, off the centerline.

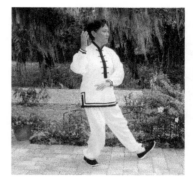

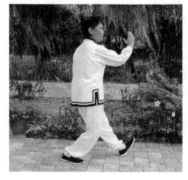

- As you slowly put 70 percent of your weight onto the left foot, the right hand pushes forward while the left hand gently moves to the front of the left hip.

- Shift your weight back onto the right leg. Turn your left foot outward, and slightly turn your body to the left.

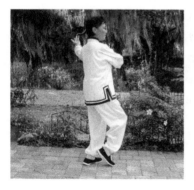

- Shift your weight onto your left leg, and bring your right foot next to the left foot. As you bring your right foot in, move the left arm downward to the left slightly behind your body to shoulder level. The right arm circles inward to chest level.

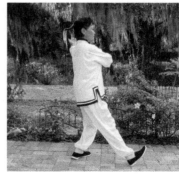

- Then step forward with your right foot, heel first, off the centerline.

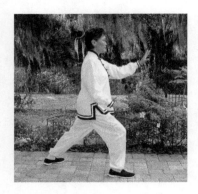

■ As you slowly put 70 percent of your weight onto the right foot, the left hand pushes forward, and the right hand gently moves to the front of the right hip.

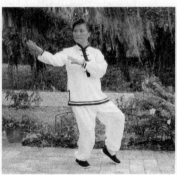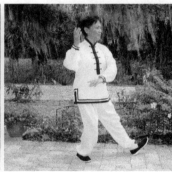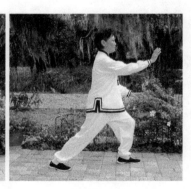

■ Repeat movement. Shift your weight back to the left leg. Turn outward with your right foot, heel down. As you bring your left foot next to the right foot, move your right arm downward to the right side slightly behind your body to shoulder level. The left arm circles inward to chest level. Then step forward with the left foot, heel down, off the centerline. As you slowly put 70 percent of your weight onto your left foot, the right hand pushes forward, and the left hand gently moves to the front of the left hip.

WEEK 4

5. PLAY GUITAR

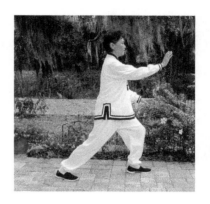

- Brush knee ends at a left lunge position. Continue to put weight on the left leg.

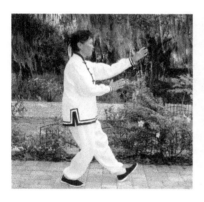

- The right foot steps forward to just slightly behind the left foot. Put your weight on the right foot. At the same time, move your right arm down to the middle of the abdomen, the fingers point forward and upward. Move the left hand upward in front of the right hand but higher. The fingers of the left hand point forward and upward, and the forearm is about heart level. Put the left heel in front of the right foot. You are now in sit-back stance.

6. STEP BACK, ROLL BACK ARMS (ALSO CALLED REPULSE THE MONKEY)

- Start from the end of play guitar.

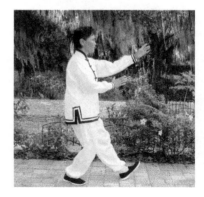

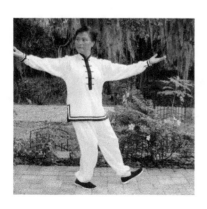

- Relax, and move the right arm back to shoulder level about 135 degrees from the left arm.

- Next lift the left leg, and at the same time, bring the right hand close to the right ear.

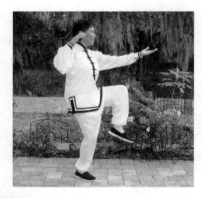

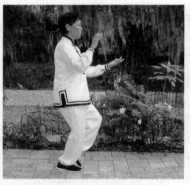

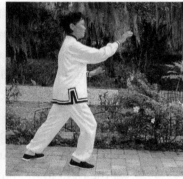

- Step back with the left leg, stepping slightly off the centerline.

- Shift your weight onto the left leg. At the same time, the right hand pushes forward, and the left hand slides back under the right arm until it reaches shoulder level, 135 degrees from the right arm. You will need to adjust the right foot to be natural. Your weight is mostly on the left, palms facing up.

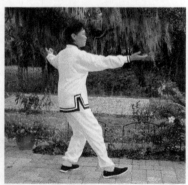

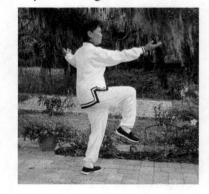

- Lift your right foot, and at the same time, bring the left hand close to the left ear.

■ Step back with the right leg, stepping slightly off the centerline. Shift your weight to the right leg, and at the same time, the left hand pushes forward, and the right hand slides back under the left arm until shoulder level, 135 degrees from the left arm. You will need to adjust the left foot to be natural. Most of your weight is on the right, palms facing up.

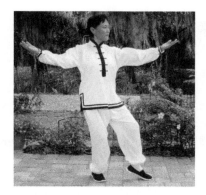

Repeat the above movements until your weight is on your right leg, palms facing up, elbows pointing down.

Week 5

1. Practice the warm-up exercises.

2. Practice taiji qigong.

3. Review taiji movements 1–6.

4. Learn movements 7–9 of the form:

   7. Grasp the bird's tail, on the left

   8. Grasp the bird's tail, on the right

   9. Single whip

5. Perform the taiji movements from 1 to 9 three times.

7. GRASP THE BIRD'S TAIL, ON THE LEFT

- Start from the end of step back, roll back arms (repulse the monkey).

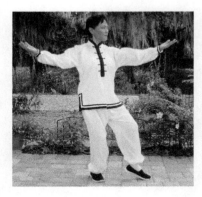

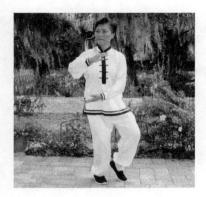

- The weight is on your right foot. Move your left hand under the right arm like you're holding a ball on your right side. Bring the left foot close to the right foot.

■ Step to the left, heel first. As you shift your weight to the left leg, move your left hand to the left at upper chest or neck level, elbow slightly bent and relaxed. Move the right hand next to the right hip.

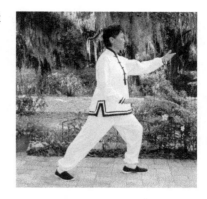

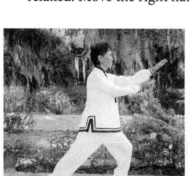

■ Move your right hand across the body to under your left wrist, palms facing each other.

■ Shift your weight to the right leg. Move both arms down and then to the right until the fingers are at eye level.

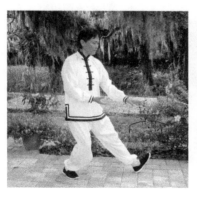

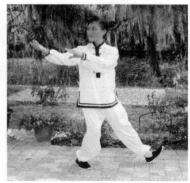

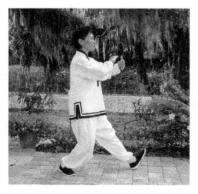

■ Shift your weight, and turn your body to the left. Move both hands to the left in front of the chest, palms facing each other like you are holding a small ball in front of your chest. You are facing left.

■ Shift your weight to the left leg.

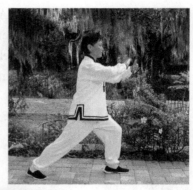

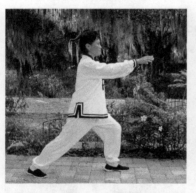

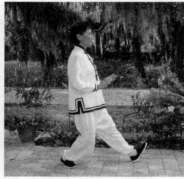

■ Open your palms, which should face down. Sit back. Your arms and hands will naturally move close to your waist.

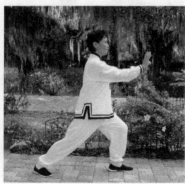

■ Shift weight to the left leg. Push the palms forward, with elbows slightly bent.

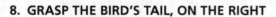

8. GRASP THE BIRD'S TAIL, ON THE RIGHT

■ Start from the end of grasp the bird's tail, on the left.

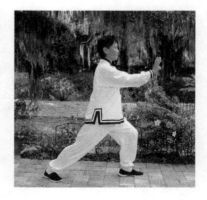

- Shift your weight enough to turn your left foot toward the right. Turn to the right, and then shift all your weight back to the left leg.

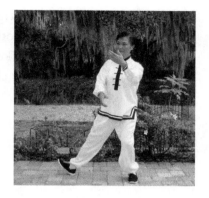

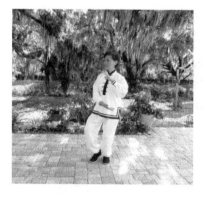

- Bring the right foot close to the left foot. Your hands are holding an imaginary ball on the left with the right hand under the left forearm.

- Step to right with your right foot, and as you are shifting weight to the right foot, move the right hand to shoulder level. At the same time, your left hand gently presses down in front of the left hip.

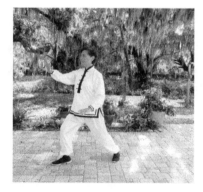

- Move the left hand across the front of the body to under the right wrist, palms facing each other.

Shift your weight to the left. Move both arms to the left until the fingers of the left hand are at eye level.

- Shift your weight to your right leg, and turn your body to the right. Move both hands to the right, palms facing each other like you're holding a small ball in front of your chest. You are now facing right.

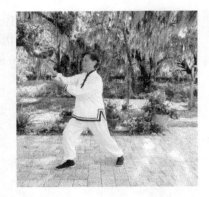

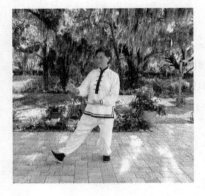

- Shift your weight back to the left foot (sit back), and bring both hands to your dan tian (lower abdomen), palms facing down.

- Shift your weight to the right. Push your palms forward (to the right), elbows slightly bent.

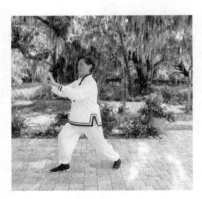

9. SINGLE WHIP

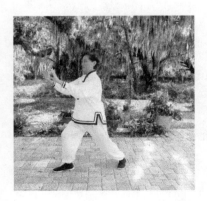

- Start from the end of grasp the bird's tail, right.

- Shift and turn to the left, then shift and turn to the right.

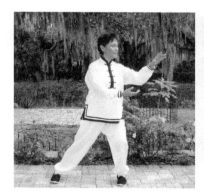 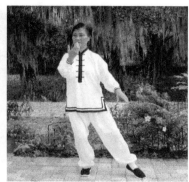

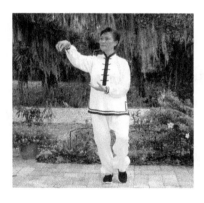

- Bring the left foot close to the right foot. At the same time, the arms follow the body from left to right. The right wrist turns downward, and all the fingers together point down. The left hand follows the body until it comes to the front of the lower abdomen, palm up.

- The left foot steps to the left. As you shift your weight to the left, your left arm follows the body to the left, and the palm moves to shoulder level, palm forward.

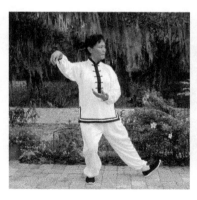 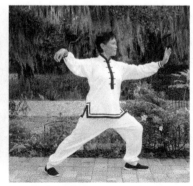

Week 6

1. Practice the warm-up exercises.

2. Practice taiji qigong.

3. Review taiji movements 1–9.

4. Learn movements 10–12 of the form:
    10. Wave hands like clouds
    11. Single whip
    12. Gauge the height of the horse (high pat on horse)

5. Perform the taiji movements from 1 to 12 three times.

10. WAVE HANDS LIKE CLOUDS

This is one of the more difficult movements in the taiji form. Remember to allow your hands to follow your body. Relax and feel for the flow. You can do it.

- Start from the single whip position, still facing left.

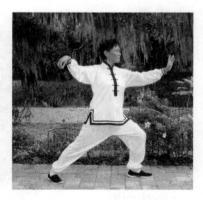

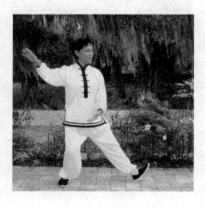

- Shift your weight to the right.

- The left arm moves downward, following the body to the right. At the same time, relax your right hand.

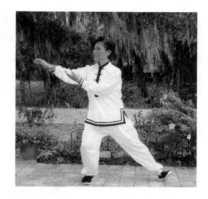

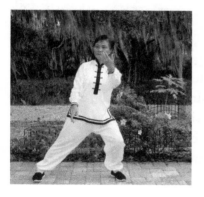

- Shift your weight to the left.

- Move your left hand to the left following the body. At the same time, the right hand waves downward, then to the left.

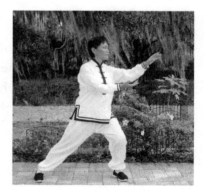

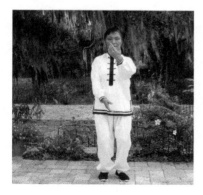

- Move your right foot close to the left foot (about one fist apart).

- Put your weight on your right foot. At the same time, the right hand waves to the right, crossing in front of the chest. The left hand waves to the right, crossing the front of the lower abdomen.

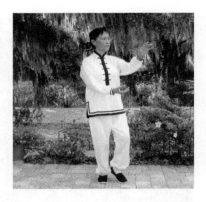

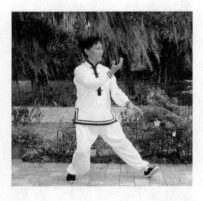

- Step to the left. The left hand (arm) waves upward and to the left, crossing in front of the chest, following the body. The right hand waves downward and to the left, crossing in front of the lower abdomen. At the same time, bring the right foot close to the left foot, spaced about one fist apart.

- Put weight on the right foot. At the same time, the right hand waves to the right, crossing in front of the chest. The left hand waves to the right, crossing in front of the lower abdomen.

11. SINGLE WHIP

Single whip occurs twice in this taiji sequence. This is the second occurrence.

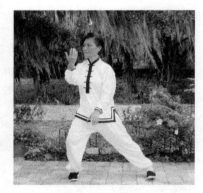

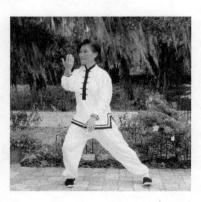

- Start from the end of wave hands like clouds.

- Shift your weight to your right leg, and bring the left foot next to the right. At the same time, turn the right wrist and hand downward. Put the five fingers together, pointing downward. The hand is about at shoulder level, toward the back of the body, about 135 degrees from the left shoulder, the elbow slightly bent. The left hand is in front of the lower abdomen, or slightly under right wrist.

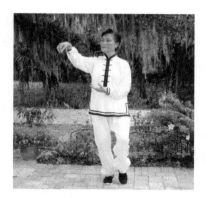

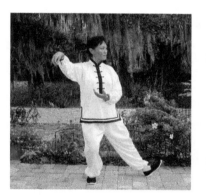

- Step to the left. Move the left hand (arm) to the left, crossing in front of the chest, following the weight as it shifts to the left. The right palm is at shoulder level. You will need to adjust the right foot to put the body in a more natural position.

- Next put 70 percent of your weight onto the left leg and 30 percent on the right leg. Your arms extend outward at about shoulder level into a very nice open position.

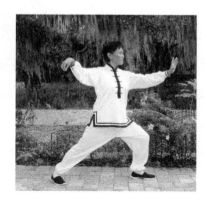

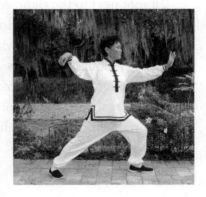

12. GAUGE THE HEIGHT OF THE HORSE (HIGH PAT ON HORSE)

- Start from the end of single whip.

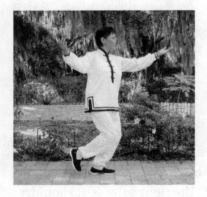

- Shift to put more weight on your left leg. Bring your right foot a half step closer to the left foot.

- Place the left toe in front of the right foot. The right palm pushes forward. The left palm withdraws to waist level. This is an empty stance.

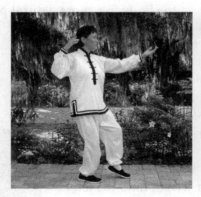

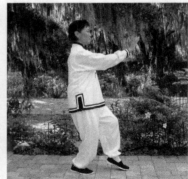

Week 7

1. Practice the warm-up exercises.

2. Practice taiji qigong.

3. Review taiji movements 1–12.

4. Learn movements 13–15 of the form:

   13. Right kick

   14. Strike the ear with fist

   15. Turn body and left kick

5. Perform the taiji movements from 1 to 15 four times.

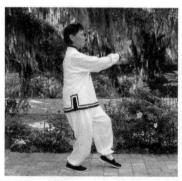

13. RIGHT KICK

- Start from the final position of gauge the height of the horse.

- Draw the right hand back to the front of the chest. Move the left hand forward above the right hand. Then both hands circle forward, upward, sideward, and downward until they reach the front of the chest.

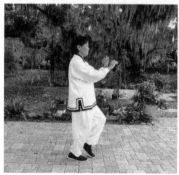
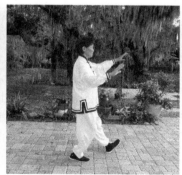

- At the same time, shift your weight to the left, and lift your right foot.

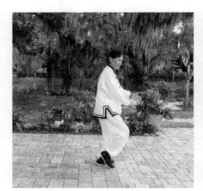

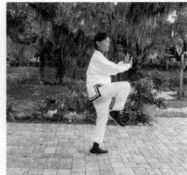

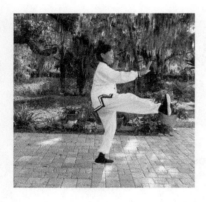

- Open both hands to the sides but at less than 180 degrees. At the same time, kick with the right foot (focus on heel) forward and slightly to the right.

14. STRIKE THE EAR WITH FIST

- Start from the end of the right kick movement.

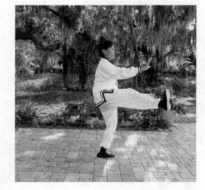

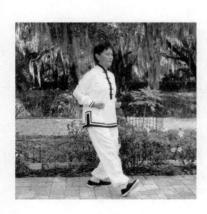

- Bring back the right foot, and land with the heel pointing in the same direction as the kick. At the same time, place both hands on the waist, making fists. Your weight is still on your left foot.

■ Shift your weight to your right foot. At the same time, move your arms outward, then to the front at temple level six inches from fist to fist. Your weight is now on your right foot.

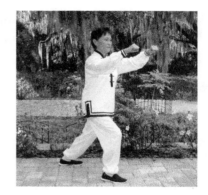

15. TURN BODY AND LEFT KICK

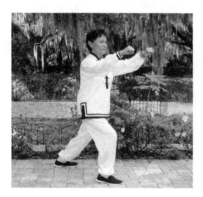

■ Start from the end of strike the ear with fist.

■ Shift your weight back to the left leg.

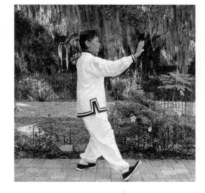

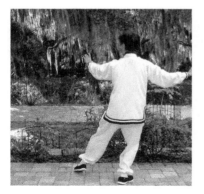

■ Turn your body to the left, and open your arms to the sides. Shift all your weight to the right leg.

- Move your arms downward, then to the front of the chest, and lift your left leg.

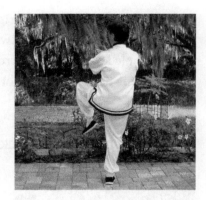

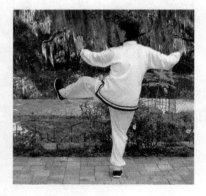

- Open both hands to the side but less than 180 degrees. At the same time, kick forward diagonally with the left foot, focusing on the heel.

Week 8

1. Practice the warm-up exercises.

2. Practice taiji thirteen movements.

3. Practice taiji qigong.

4. Review taiji movement 1–15.

5. Learn movements 16–18 of the form:
   16. Left low stance, stand on left leg (snake creeping down, golden pheasant standing on left leg)
   17. Right low stance, stand on right leg (snake creeping down, golden pheasant standing on right leg)
   18. Move the shuttle, left then right (fair lady moves the shuttle)

6. Perform the taiji movements from 1 to 18 three times.

16. LEFT LOW STANCE, STAND ON LEFT LEG (SNAKE CREEPING DOWN, GOLDEN PHEASANT STANDING ON LEFT LEG)

This is the most difficult movement. Beginners often have trouble with it. But once you let the body go with the flow, you will do well. Keep in mind that the harder you try, the worse you get. This is the Dao (the Way). When you go with the Dao, the process of learning taiji is much easier and more relaxed—plus, you obtain more benefits.

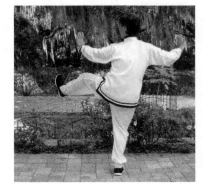

- Start from the end of the turn body and left kick movement.

- After the left kick, bring the left leg back, and put it down to restore your balance. At the same time, place both hands to the right with the left palm open and turned upward and the right-hand fingers together and pointing downward.

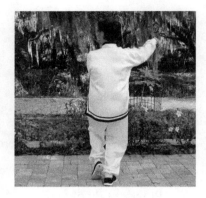

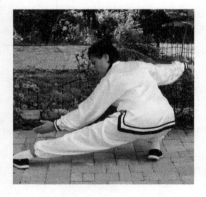

- Take a big step to the left diagonally. Move your left hand downward and leftward along the left leg.

- Turn the left foot to the left, and face left. Shift your weight to your left leg. At the same time, move your left hand upward, and move your right hand downward. The five fingers of the right hand are still held together, facing upward.

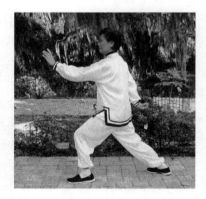

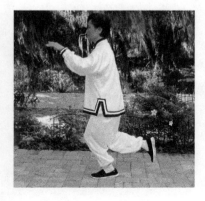

- Continue to shift your weight to the left, and lift your right leg.

- At the same time, your left hand moves downward, palm pressing down.

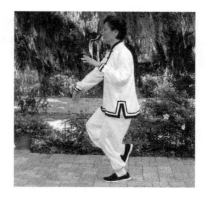

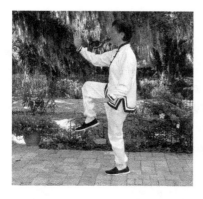

- The right hand moves downward, then upward. Sink your palm with the fingers now open and pointing upward in front of your body while the left hand is near your hip, palm down. You are now standing on your left leg.

17. RIGHT LOW STANCE, STAND ON RIGHT LEG (SNAKE CREEPING DOWN, GOLDEN PHEASANT STANDING ON RIGHT LEG)

- Start from the end of the left low stance, stand on left leg movement.

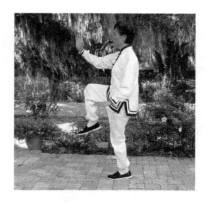

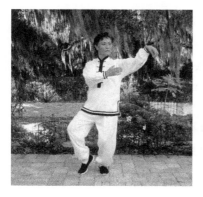

- Put down your right foot. Turn your body to face front. Your weight is still on the left leg. At the same time, place both hands to the left with the right palm open and turned upward and the left-hand fingers together and pointing downward.

- Take a big step to the right diagonally. Move your right hand downward and rightward along the right leg.

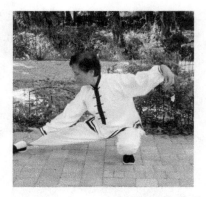

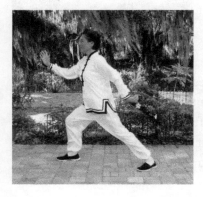

- Turn the right foot to the right, and face right. Shift your weight to your right leg. At the same time, move your right hand upward, and move your left hand downward. The five fingers of the left hand are still together, facing upward.

- Continue to shift your weight to your right leg, and lift your left leg.

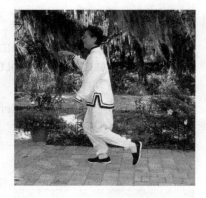

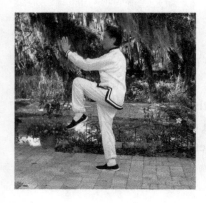

- The right hand moves downward with the palm pressing down. The left hand moves downward, then upward. Sink your palm with the fingers now open and pointing upward in front of the body while the right hand is near your hip, palm down. You are now standing on your right leg.

18. MOVE THE SHUTTLE, LEFT THEN RIGHT (FAIR LADY MOVES THE SHUTTLE)

- Start from the end of right low stance.

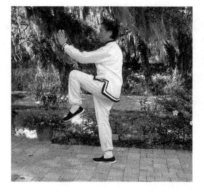

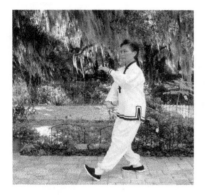

- Your left foot steps down diagonally toward your left. The arms naturally gather in front of the body, like holding a ball in front of the body.

- Shift your weight to the left foot. Bring your right foot close to your left foot.

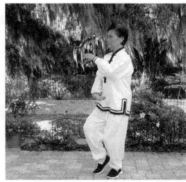

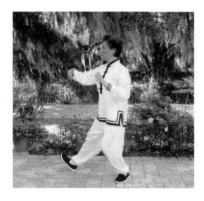

- Then step out diagonally to your right.

- At the same time, the left hand pushes forward, and the right hand moves upward, above the right temple. You should feel like you are blocking and redirecting an incoming force with your right arm.

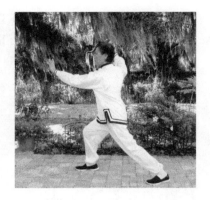

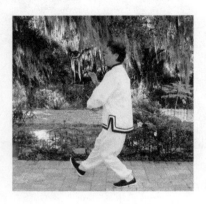

- Shift your weight back onto the left foot. Your arms naturally gather in front of the body, like holding a ball in front of the body.

- Shift your weight to the right foot, and bring the left foot close to the right foot.

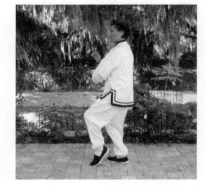

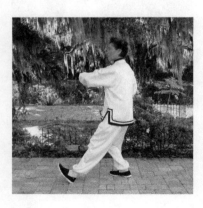

- Next step out diagonally to your left.

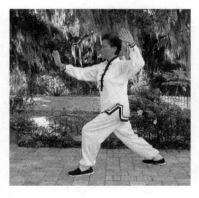

- At same time, your right hand pushes forward, and the left hand moves upward, above the left temple. You should feel like you are blocking and redirecting an incoming force with your left arm.

Week 9

1. Practice the warm-up exercises.

2. Practice taiji thirteen movements.

3. Practice taiji qigong.

4. Review taiji movements 1–18.

5. Learn movements 19–21 of the form:
   19. Pick needle from the sea
   20. Send a flash through the arms
   21. Turn body, deflect, block, and punch

6. Perform the taiji movements from 1 to 21 three times.

19. PICK NEEDLE FROM THE SEA

■ Start from the end of the move the shuttle
movement.

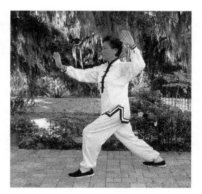

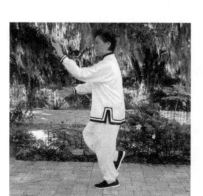

■ Bring your right foot a half step closer but still
behind your left foot, and move your left hand to
the front of your body, and lower your right hand.

- Then put your weight on the right foot, and slightly lift your left foot. At the same time, continue moving your right hand downward, and then bring it backward. Move your left hand downward.

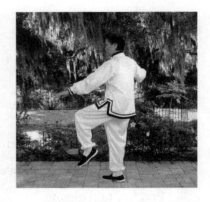

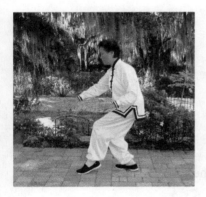

- Lower the left leg so the toes gently touch the ground (your weight is still on your right leg). At the same time, move your right hand downward and forward with the fingers pointing 45 degrees downward in front of the body. Your upper body is slightly forward.

20. SEND A FLASH THROUGH THE ARMS

- Start from the end of pick needle from the sea.

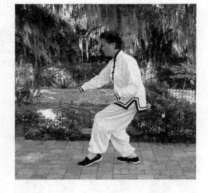

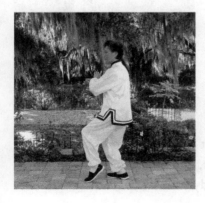

- Bring the left foot a little closer to the right foot. Gather both hands in front of the chest.

- Step out with the left foot. As you shift your weight onto the left foot, move the left arm to your left with open palm. The right arm moves above the head with open palm. Look at the left hand.

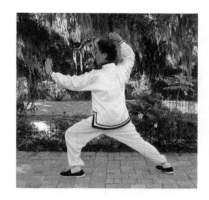

21. TURN BODY, DEFLECT, BLOCK, AND PUNCH

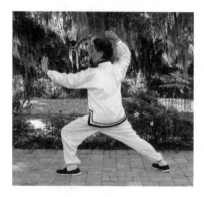

- Start from the end of send a flash through the arms.

- Shift your weight, and turn your body to the right. Move the left toes inward and the right toes outward. At the same time, move your right arm to shoulder level, and turn the left palm to face up.

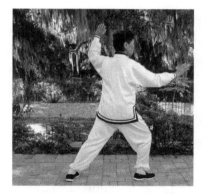

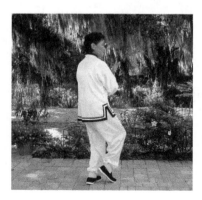

- Shift your weight to the left foot. Move the right palm downward to the front of the body, and make a fist. At the same time, move the left hand slightly upward, then to the front of the chest, palm facing down. Bring the right foot close to the left foot.

■ The right foot steps out to the right, heel first. The right fist moves upward and forward.

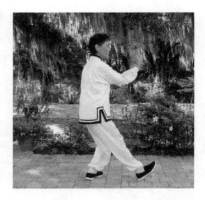

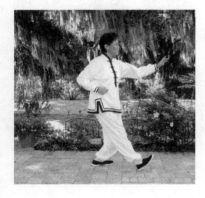

■ Put weight on the right leg, and turn your body to the right. The right arm follows the body and circles to the right. Make a gentle fist with your right hand, and move it to your waist. The left hand follows the body until it is in front of the body in guard position.

■ The left foot steps forward, heel first.

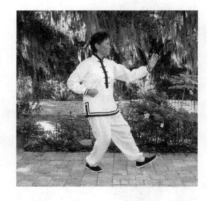

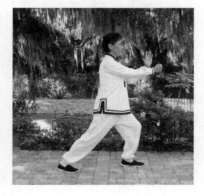

■ As you shift your weight onto your left leg, move the right fist forward at chest level. The left hand is still in guard position, next to the right forearm.

Week 10

1. Practice the warm-up exercises.

2. Practice taiji thirteen movements.

3. Practice taiji qigong.

4. Review taiji movements 1–21.

5. Learn movements 22–24 of the form:
   22. Pull back, then push
   23. Cross hands
   24. Taiji ending, closing position

6. Perform the taiji movements from 1 to 24 three times.

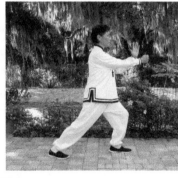

22. PULL BACK, THEN PUSH

- Start from the end of turn body, deflect, block, and punch.

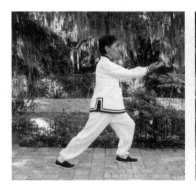

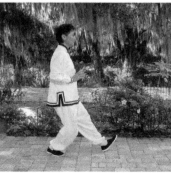

- Open your palms, and shift your weight back to the right leg. Both hands follow the body.

- Shift your weight forward onto the left leg, and push the palms forward until the arms are slightly bent.

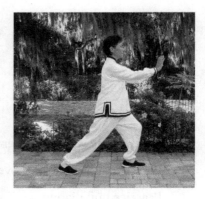

23. CROSS HANDS

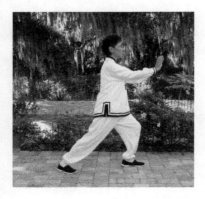

- Start from the push palm position.

- Turn the right foot rightward about 90 degrees and the left foot inward toward the front. At the same time, shift your weight to the right, and move your right arm to the right at shoulder level.

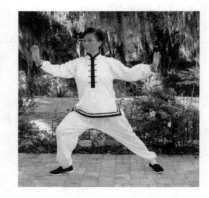

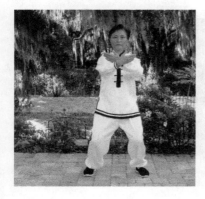

- Shift your weight to the left, and bring the right foot next to the left foot. The feet are shoulder width apart and face forward. At the same time, bring both arms to the front of the chest, crossing wrists with right hand in front of the left hand. You are now in horse stance with knees and lower back relaxed.

24. TAIJI ENDING, CLOSING POSITION

- Start from the end of cross hands.

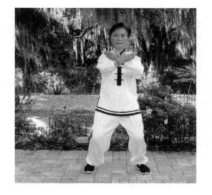

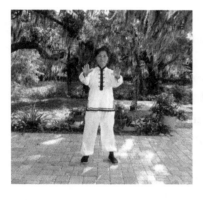

- Inhale, raise your body, and open your hands in front of the chest. Slowly turn the palms to face downward. Exhale naturally while moving the arms and palms downward.

- Bring the left foot next to the right foot, and relax your entire body.

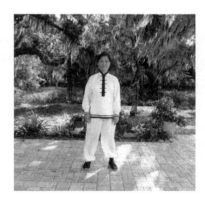

Self-Check List

- Are you able to practice twenty-four-steps taiji-quan fluidly?

- Are you familiar with Daoist philosophy and its relation to taiji?

- Are you committed to making taiji a lifetime practice?

- Did you go through all the movements and feel the energy in your hands and body?

- Do you feel calmer and have more energy after your taiji practice?

- Are you able to focus better and let go of negative thoughts in general?

- Are you ready to move to the next level? Do you want to explore the martial application of taiji, learn self-defense with taiji, or do partner taiji practice and taiji push hands?

If you answer yes to all of the above, you are ready to take yourself to the next level. You can start your level-two taiji practice, which includes learning other forms, taiji push hands, and two-person taiji practice.

With significant time and practice, you might even think about becoming an instructor to share your knowledge and skill with others. In my instructor training course, the teaching strategy is thoroughly discussed.

Taiji is a journey—a happy and a healthy journey. This journey may not have shortcuts, but it will give you joy, peace, energy, and happiness. You are not alone because there are many people in the world on the same journey; they are walking with you. Every year, on the last Saturday of April, people around the world celebrate World Tai Chi & Qigong Day. We gather in public places to practice these arts and raise world energy, natural healing, and well-being. For more information on this event, please see worldtaichiday.org. You can either join a local group or start your own and become part of this energy wave. The more we practice outdoors, the more exposure we give our art. Then people will eventually get interested in this kind of practice, learn more, and join.

I hope you have a wonderful taiji journey.

Taiji 10-Week Plan

New skills are listed in red. After a week of practice, skills are listed in **black**.
Check off each day as you move through the calendar. Have fun and relax!

Week	Daily Practice	Day 1	Day 2	Day 3	Day 4	Day 5	Day 6	Day 7
1	☐ Learn warm-up exercises ☐ Learn taiji stances ☐ Learn taiji walking ☐ Learn taiji basics	☐☐☐☐	☐☐☐☐	☐☐☐☐	☐☐☐☐	☐☐☐☐	☐☐☐☐	☐☐☐☐
2	☐ Warm-up exercises ☐ Taiji stances ☐ Taiji walking ☐ Taiji basics ☐ Learn taiji 13 movements	☐☐☐☐ ☐	☐☐☐☐ ☐	☐☐☐☐ ☐	☐☐☐☐ ☐	☐☐☐☐ ☐	☐☐☐☐ ☐	☐☐☐☐ ☐

3	☐ Warm-up exercises
	☐ Taiji walking
	☐ Learn taiji qigong
	☐ Taiji 13 movements
	☐ Learn moves 1–3 of form:
	  1. Taiji preparation
	  2. Parting wild horse's mane
	  3. White crane spreads wings
		☐☐☐☐ ☐	☐☐☐☐ ☐	☐☐☐☐ ☐	☐☐☐☐ ☐	☐☐☐☐ ☐	☐☐☐☐ ☐	☐☐☐☐ ☐

4	☐ Warm-up exercises
	☐ Taiji basics
	☐ Taiji qigong
	☐ Taiji 13 movements
	☐ Learn moves 4–6:
	  4. Brush knee
	  5. Play guitar
	  6. Repulse monkey
	☐ Form: moves 1–6 *(3 times)*
		☐☐☐☐ ☐ ☐	☐☐☐☐ ☐ ☐	☐☐☐☐ ☐ ☐	☐☐☐☐ ☐ ☐	☐☐☐☐ ☐ ☐	☐☐☐☐ ☐ ☐	☐☐☐☐ ☐ ☐

Week	Daily Practice	Day 1	Day 2	Day 3	Day 4	Day 5	Day 6	Day 7
5	☐ Warm-up exercises ☐ Taiji qigong ☐ Form, moves 1–6	☐ ☐ ☐	☐ ☐ ☐	☐ ☐ ☐	☐ ☐ ☐	☐ ☐ ☐	☐ ☐ ☐	☐ ☐ ☐

	☐ Learn moves 7–9:
	   7. Grasp bird's tail, left
	   8. Grasp bird's tail, right
	   9. Single whip
		☐	☐	☐	☐	☐	☐	☐

	☐ Form: moves 1–9 *(3 times)*	☐	☐	☐	☐	☐	☐	☐
6	☐ Warm-up exercises ☐ Taiji qigong ☐ Form, moves 1–9	☐ ☐ ☐	☐ ☐ ☐	☐ ☐ ☐	☐ ☐ ☐	☐ ☐ ☐	☐ ☐ ☐	☐ ☐ ☐

	☐ Learn moves 10–12:
	   10. Wave hands like clouds
	   11. Single whip
	   12. Gauge height of horse
		☐	☐	☐	☐	☐	☐	☐

	☐ Form: moves 1–12 *(3 times)*	☐	☐	☐	☐	☐	☐	☐
7	☐ Warm-up exercises ☐ Taiji qigong ☐ Form, moves 1–12	☐ ☐ ☐	☐ ☐ ☐	☐ ☐ ☐	☐ ☐ ☐	☐ ☐ ☐	☐ ☐ ☐	☐ ☐ ☐

	☐ Learn moves 13–15:
	   13. Right kick
	   14. Strike ear with fist
	   15. Turn body and left kick
		☐	☐	☐	☐	☐	☐	☐

	☐ Form: moves 1–15 *(3 times)*	☐	☐	☐	☐	☐	☐	☐

Week	Daily Practice	Day 1	Day 2	Day 3	Day 4	Day 5	Day 6	Day 7
8	☐ Warm-up exercises ☐ Taiji 13 movements ☐ Taiji qigong ☐ Form, moves 1–15	☐☐☐☐	☐☐☐☐	☐☐☐☐	☐☐☐☐	☐☐☐☐	☐☐☐☐	☐☐☐☐

	☐ Learn moves 16–18:
	  16. Snake creeps down, golden pheasant stands on left leg
	  17. Snake creeps down, golden pheasant stands on right leg
	  18. Fair lady moves shuttle
		☐	☐	☐	☐	☐	☐	☐

	☐ Form: moves 1–18 *(3 times)*	☐	☐	☐	☐	☐	☐	☐
9	☐ Warm-up exercises ☐ Taiji 13 movements ☐ Taiji qigong ☐ Form, moves 1–18	☐☐☐☐	☐☐☐☐	☐☐☐☐	☐☐☐☐	☐☐☐☐	☐☐☐☐	☐☐☐☐

	☐ Learn moves 19–21:
	  19. Pick needle from sea
	  20. Send flash through arms
	  21. Turn body, deflect, block, and punch
		☐	☐	☐	☐	☐	☐	☐

	☐ Form: moves 1–21 *(3 times)*	☐	☐	☐	☐	☐	☐	☐
10	☐ Warm-up exercises ☐ Taiji 13 movements ☐ Taiji qigong ☐ Form, moves 1–21	☐☐☐☐	☐☐☐☐	☐☐☐☐	☐☐☐☐	☐☐☐☐	☐☐☐☐	☐☐☐☐

	☐ Learn moves 22–24:
	  22. Pull back, then push
	  23. Cross hands
	  24. Taiji ending
		☐	☐	☐	☐	☐	☐	☐

	☐ Form: moves 1–24 *(3 times)*	☐	☐	☐	☐	☐	☐	☐

Letters from Students

My fourteen-year-old son has been taking taiji classes with you for the past six months. I want you to know how much he has benefited from your classes. You have truly been an inspiration through your guidance and encouragement. He has gained a strong feeling of accomplishment and has improved his self-esteem from learning the art of taiji. In addition, it gives him a sense of inner peace and calmness that he did not have before.

—Valerie M., Bellingham, Massachusetts

I am a seventy-two-year-old woman who has been participating in weekly taiji classes from you, Dr. Kuhn. Specific benefits that I have experienced are increased vitality and flexibility, resulting in fewer aches and pains that are a part of the aging process. It is wonderful to seldom have back pain or a headache. Very important stress reduction for me has occurred naturally, creating physical and mental harmony. I would recommend your taiji classes for anyone of any age, especially the elderly.

—Naomi A., Milford, Massachusetts

Dear Dr. Kuhn,

I am so pleased with the results of my daily taiji practice. I have made so many quality improvements in my health, my brain, my emotions, and consequently, my life! I know that if I continue to practice my taiji daily, I will stay healthy.

—Gloria D., Hopedale, Massachusetts

I started my taiji/qigong exploration in January 2003, at fifty-one years of age.

The random fitness efforts I was engaged in were not producing a stable state of well-being. My energy level was up and down in big swings, even during the course of a single day. I was recovering from a frozen shoulder with physical therapy but felt like age was catching up with me. I was also presenting symptoms of liver disease, due to a fatty liver. I enjoyed benefits from a meditation practice but also recognized that life is an exploration of mind, body, and spirit. My mind-body connection

189

was sending out an SOS for help. After reading some information on taiji healing, I decided I would get involved in taiji practice. Patience, persistence, controlled relaxation, along with breathing in and with the flow of qi provided me with a wide range of healing. My energy level is now most often on an even keel, the symptoms of fatty liver have been relieved, and my range of motion has improved dramatically. There are multiple taiji forms and qigong exercises that provide great benefits. Your sixteen-step taiji form is where I find my greatest balance. Its design promotes harmony of thought and a deeply rooted sense of well-being. The sixteen-step form incorporates all the elements, and benefits, of basic taiji practice. With patience, one begins to gradually add synchronization of breathing with the movements of the form. The combination invokes a level of relaxation that I have only achieved previously during meditation. This in combination with improving balance, lower body strength, and range of motion has helped me feel younger and more optimistic in maintaining an active and healthy lifestyle now and into the years ahead. Thank you, many times over, to Dr. Aihan Kuhn, the New England School of Tai Chi, Chinese Medicine for Health, Inc., and all the gifted and talented instructors and healing practitioners.

—Larry J.

I have been practicing taiji in your school for four years now and plan on continuing my practice for the next hundred years. At first, learning taiji was confusing for me. I kept worrying about which foot should be in front or where my hands should be and any number of details. The taiji movements felt a little awkward because I still hadn't learned how to move in a natural, relaxed way. Relaxation was something that I was not used to doing in my fast-paced, high-stress career; however, with some time and patience, I found that my body was improving physically. I was becoming more flexible and more balanced. Once I learned to relax in my taiji practice, the movements started to make sense, and I was able to very quickly learn the basics about many different taiji forms. One thing that surprised me was that I found that I was able to cope with the day-to-day stresses and problems that everyone encounters every day without the aggravation and stress that I used to experience before learning taiji. After continued practice and learning the various skills and techniques, and most of all learning to relax, I found that the same improvements in flexibility and balance were happening to me mentally, affecting my personal and business relationships for the better. In the end I learned that taiji is a great way to exercise your body and your mind. Thank you, Aihan.

—Jim A.

Dear Dr. Kuhn,

Here is my story of how taiji has made a difference in my life. It is a bit long in the telling, but you can certainly take from it as much or as little as you wish to take.

I studied taiji sixteen steps with Dr. Aihan Kuhn from September 2005 through May 2006. The results of this practice have amazed me! I offer the following two examples of what taiji practice has accomplished in my life.

After the very first taiji class, I felt a reconnection between the two sides of my head. There had been a very, very slight feeling of disconnection for the twenty-six years prior—this manifestation had occurred as a reaction to an ear infection and was made worse by an extremely stressful life event. No doctor except a chiropractor had ever been able to improve this situation, and the correction was only temporary even with chiropractic. After only one taiji class, the problem disappeared.

A few weeks after beginning sixteen-step taiji practice, I found myself saying one day, "My joy has returned." Although I had spent the previous nine years giving attention and care to three elderly relatives, then experiencing their deaths, living under conditions that were less than comfortable, and working at a demanding job, my natural joy returned. Nothing in my life except taiji practice was different. My life situation was the same as it had been for many years—only taiji practice had been added, and that made all the difference.

I realized that for as long as I could remember—and that is many years, as I am now a grandmother—I had to work at bringing up and keeping a joyful attitude; now, it is no effort at all—it happens on its own. I am convinced, and I will continue my taiji journey.

My best to you and your family.

—Elaine B., Massachusetts

Testimonials from the Tai Chi Instructor Training Program

Dr. Kuhn, your studio has been our second home this year—a taiji qigong vacation. I loved your guidance and really enjoyed this taiji training class. Thank you, thank you, and thank you.

—Tom B., Minnesota

It was an awesome class! I learned a lot! I hope you do some intensive class for us in the near future, to learn more details and martial applications.

—Pam A., New Jersey

I have taken several taiji training classes. But your ability to explain every detail is excellent. Therefore, I learn more in detail. I loved it!

—John D., Massachusetts

Excellent job! Taiji should be mandatory in school. I feel so much better besides learning.

—Cynthia S., New York

Thank you, Dr. Kuhn, for your outstanding wisdom, your concerns for my health, and your effort in teaching the forms with integrity according to the tradition. Thank you for teaching taiji to a deeper degree by incorporating the gathering of inner qi. You are an amazing person. Thank you again. I am looking forward to seeing you again very soon.

—Dorothy A., Chicago, Illinois

I drove eight hours to come to this training. I realized it was well worth the trip. Your training is well organized, pleasant, and really foundation building. It helps a lot! I look forward to do more training with you soon! Thank you!

—Jean L., Georgia

Everything is so positive in your training. I loved it! I learned a lot more than expected—you taught us more than just learning a taiji form. You are a great teacher, great environment.

—Zac W., Massachusetts

Excellent class! Dr. Kuhn is wonderful! Driving ten hours is worth the trip to spend time as her student. Feel very honored to call her my teacher. Thank you so much. This is a life-changing experience for me.

—Denise J., Maryland

Excellent class! It was exactly what I wanted! Three days is intense but needed to get the basics and basic forms. The warm-up and stretching is helpful, and I really appreciated you explaining the health benefits from doing taiji. I recommend this training to anyone. Even a person who has no experience can benefit.

—Lisa Z., Illinois

Of all the years I have been searching in the martial arts . . . Dr. Kuhn answered many of the questions I had but could not get answered. She is wise and generous with her knowledge; she is warm and welcoming. I learned with ease. Thank you so much for giving and sharing. I will be continuing to learn from you.

—Mark C., New Hampshire

I would love for the class to last longer. Dr. Kuhn has amazing energy. She has so much patience as a teacher. She really cares about her students and gives them the skills and the tools they need to go out and teach others this healing art form.

—Sandra D., Georgia

Dr. Kuhn, I truly appreciated your patience. You are a skilled teacher. The way you broke down complex moves into simple steps really helped. Your positive attitude was really motivating when I felt stuck.

—Eileen F., Georgia

I would love to see you offer a weeklong training for both parts of taiji.

—Ben K., Florida

Thank you, Dr. K., for a fantastic weekend learning taiji! I cannot wait for Tai Chi II in July. I've also started reading your book about taiji and depression. Everything you said makes perfect sense. I already have plans on how I can work that into my training and everyday life. You have made such a difference already in my life, and I can't wait to see what else we can do together. Dr. Kuhn, you are amazing!

—Kim B., Georgia

Thank you, Dr. Kuhn, for changing my life and helping me start a new taiji journey. I feel so good the entire training. It is a wonderful positive energy imparted throughout the course. Your method of teaching is so good that anyone can learn taiji from the way you teach.

—Jeff M.

Notes

1. Peter M. Wayne, *Harvard Medical School Guide to Tai Chi: 12 Weeks to a Healthy Body, Strong Heart, and Sharp Mind* (Boston, MA: Shambhala, 2013).

2. Michael R. Irwin, Jennifer L. Pike, Jason C. Cole, and Michael N. Oxman, "Effects of a Behavioral Intervention, Tai Chi Chih, on Varicella-Zoster Virus Specific Immunity and Health Functioning in Older Adults," *Psychosomatic Medicine* 65 (2003): 824–830. Results of the study were published in the September 2003 issue of *Psychosomatic Medicine*.

Acknowledgments

I studied taiji in medical school in China from 1977 to 1982. At the time I was just learning the movements and did not really know much about taiji. I did not make the connection between mind and body during my time in medical school. At that time I did not even understand the concept of meditation. After practicing taiji for more than thirty years and teaching it for more than twenty years, I really feel the benefits, and I am able to share taiji wisdom with others. One thing I can say with confidence is that taiji changed my life. It sharpened my intellect, made me more intuitive, and brought me many other invaluable benefits.

I was fortunate that I had the chance to learn from some of the world's greatest masters. I am so grateful that each of these masters taught me different things and gave me tips about taiji, qigong, and life.

First I worked with Grandmaster Duan Zhi Liang, who is a grandmaster of qigong and Chinese medicine. Even though at the time he was ninety-seven years old, his sense of humor was so incredible. I loved him very much. He not only taught me the qigong form but also a most important life lesson: "Treat your friends well, and also treat your enemies well. Then you will have no enemies." He is also an inspiration in my antiaging practice. Every time I think about getting older and being unable to do things I'd like to do, I think about him. I then change my thoughts: I remind myself that I can still do so many things that I love to do.

I was also very fortunate to learn from Grandmaster Feng Zhi Qiang. He was seventeenth in the lineage of Chen-style taijiquan, and he was such a nice man that anyone would love him. He treated me like a daughter. He was kind, gentle, and persuasive. Even though he was one of the best-known and strongest masters in the world, his humility really inspired me. He knew that I am a doctor of holistic medicine, and during a visit to Beijing, I treated him for a neck problem. I felt like I was treating my father. The way he talked was like my father too. The second time I visited him in Beijing, he called me Monkey. Not only because I was born in the year of the monkey, but also because he thought that I was a faster learner, a "monkey student." I knew I had to work hard in order to please him because the world respects him so much. He passed in 2012, and I cried when I heard the news. I love him so much, and I really miss him. I also know I still have so much to learn.

The biggest lesson I learned from Grandmaster Feng Zhi Qiang was about real relaxation. I learned that no matter how well you execute the form, you can't get the maximum benefit until you learn to relax. Being with him, I felt very comfortable and relaxed. No one dared to joke in front of him like I did, but he laughed and understood my sense of humor.

I then had several chances to work with Grandmaster Li De Ying. He was vice-chairman of the Chinese Martial Art Committee and a professor at the Martial Art Department of the Beijing People's University. He is so knowledgeable and really helped me with the theory, history, and philosophy of martial art and taiji. This is how I came to understand the "how and why" things work, how and why we should practice correctly. So now I am able to share with my students and pass the knowledge on to the next generation of instructors. He was so amazed that I was not trained in martial art to begin with but rather trained in the medical field. But he knew that my passion and my dedication to the work would bring good results in my learning and teaching. He told me my students showed that they had a good foundation, which made me very happy. The best part of learning with him was his "theory of everything."

I also had several chances to learn with Grandmaster Zhu Tian Cai. He is also in the lineage of the Chen-style taijiquan masters. He is a very nice man, easygoing, and pleasant to be with. Learning push-hands from him, I gained not only the techniques but also the theory and teaching methods. The lesson I learned from him is to teach with passion. Teach whatever you can to help students improve, and don't just teach partially, as many masters do. Grandmaster Zhu Tian Cai has incredible energy. He is strong on both a physical and an emotional level. I feel relaxed being with him. This has made me more aware that I need to find ways to make my students feel relaxed when they are with me.

I learned from several other masters too, including masters who taught me bagua, xingyi, Chen-style taiji, and other forms. Every one of them has something unique and special to offer. Some things they have in common are they are all very kind, easygoing, and open minded. They teach in a persuasive way, not a critical way. They all have amazing moral character, are sincere, are strong emotionally, have mental clarity, and have a lot of life's wisdom.

I am very grateful, and I appreciate everything they taught me. I feel so fortunate to have had them in my life. I am also grateful that I have so many wonderful students. I will continue to share with my students all of the knowledge and wisdom that my masters have taught me. And I hope that we can all help to pass this valuable knowledge to the next generation.

About the Author

Dr. Aihan Kuhn is a unique doctor of natural medicine (holistic medicine). She is a speaker, an award-winning author, and a master of taiji and qigong. Trained in both conventional medicine and traditional Chinese medicine, Dr. Kuhn has helped thousands of patients overcome various physical ailments and emotional imbalances. She incorporates taiji and qigong into her healing methodologies, changing the lives of people who had struggled for many years and had no relief from conventional 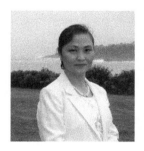 medicine. From her healing, patients also learn self-care techniques and strategies that help them to continue their healing journey at home. These techniques also help self-confidence, relationships, stress management, daily energy level, and better focus.

Dr. Kuhn provides many wellness programs, natural healing workshops, and professional training programs, such as her Tai Chi Instructor Training, Qi Gong Instructor Training, and Wellness Tui Na Therapy certification courses. These highly rated programs have produced many quality teachers and therapists.

Dr. Kuhn is president of the Tai Chi & Qi Gong Healing Institute (www.TaiChi-Healing.org), which is a nonprofit organization that promotes natural healing and prevention through an annual natural healing conference, World Tai Chi Day, healing qigong exercises, Daoist study, and special programs.

Dr. Kuhn now lives in Sarasota, Florida. She continues her natural healing education and offers consultations and private healing retreats for people who live far away to help them restore their health, inner balance, and vitality. For more information, please visit her website, www.draihankuhn.com.

Dr. Kuhn offers wellness education programs to help people improve their health, career, and overall quality of life. These programs include the following:

- The Secrets to Women's Health and Healing
- Natural Methods for Relief from Anxiety
- The Road to Fearless Living
- Relieve Stress in Seven Minutes
- Medicine: East Meets West
- Lose Weight in Seven Days
- Cancer Healing the Natural Way
- Weight Loss the Natural Way
- Qigong for Your Brain
- Emotion Healing through Body Movements
- Brain Fitness
- Food and Healing

Professional Training Programs (all offer continuing education credits for massage therapists):
- Qi Gong Instructor Training
- Tai Chi Instructor Training
- Wellness Tui Na Therapy
- Tui Na for Back Therapy
- Tui Na for Neck Therapy

For more information,

please visit www.DrAihanKuhn.com and

www.taichihealing.org.

Books by Dr. Kuhn:

Simple Chinese Medicine

Natural Healing with Qigong

Tai Chi for Depression

Weight Loss the Natural Way

Qi Gong for Travelers

   Tai Chi in 10 Weeks

   Brain Fitness

Videos by Dr. Kuhn::

Tai Chi Chuan (24 Steps, Yang Style)
Tai Chi Chuan (42 Steps, Combined Style)
Tai Chi Chuan (24 Steps, Chen Style)
Tai Chi Sward (42 Steps, Combined Style)
Tai Chi Fan (Single Fan)
Tai Chi 16 Steps (for Internal Healing)
Therapeutic Qi Gong (36 Movements)
Meridian Qi Gong
Qi Gong for Arthritis
Circle Energy Qi Gong
Eight Brocade Qi Gong
Twelve Minutes Qi Gong for Computer Users
Tai Chi for Depression
Dr. Kuhn Tai Chi Form Collection

6 HEALING MOVEMENTS
101 REFLECTIONS ON TAI CHI CHUAN
108 INSIGHTS INTO TAI CHI CHUAN
ADVANCING IN TAE KWON DO
ANALYSIS OF SHAOLIN CHIN NA 2ND ED
ANCIENT CHINESE WEAPONS
THE ART AND SCIENCE OF STAFF FIGHTING
ART OF HOJO UNDO
ARTHRITIS RELIEF, 3D ED.
BACK PAIN RELIEF, 2ND ED.
BAGUAZHANG, 2ND ED.
BRAIN FITNESS
CARDIO KICKBOXING ELITE
CHIN NA IN GROUND FIGHTING
CHINESE FAST WRESTLING
CHINESE FITNESS
CHINESE TUI NA MASSAGE
CHOJUN
COMPREHENSIVE APPLICATIONS OF SHAOLIN CHIN NA
CONFLICT COMMUNICATION
CROCODILE AND THE CRANE: A NOVEL
CUTTING SEASON: A XENON PEARL MARTIAL ARTS THRILLER
DEFENSIVE TACTICS
DESHI: A CONNOR BURKE MARTIAL ARTS THRILLER
DIRTY GROUND
DR. WU'S HEAD MASSAGE
DUKKHA HUNGRY GHOSTS
DUKKHA REVERB
DUKKHA, THE SUFFERING: AN EYE FOR AN EYE
DUKKHA UNLOADED
ENZAN: THE FAR MOUNTAIN, A CONNOR BURKE MARTIAL
    ARTS THRILLER
ESSENCE OF SHAOLIN WHITE CRANE
EXPLORING TAI CHI
FACING VIOLENCE
FIGHT BACK
FIGHT LIKE A PHYSICIST
THE FIGHTER'S BODY
FIGHTER'S FACT BOOK
FIGHTER'S FACT BOOK 2
FIGHTING THE PAIN RESISTANT ATTACKER
FIRST DEFENSE
FORCE DECISIONS: A CITIZENS GUIDE
FOX BORROWS THE TIGER'S AWE
INSIDE TAI CHI
KAGE: THE SHADOW, A CONNOR BURKE MARTIAL ARTS
    THRILLER
KATA AND THE TRANSMISSION OF KNOWLEDGE
KRAV MAGA PROFESSIONAL TACTICS
KRAV MAGA WEAPON DEFENSES
LITTLE BLACK BOOK OF VIOLENCE
LIUHEBAFA FIVE CHARACTER SECRETS
MARTIAL ARTS ATHLETE
MARTIAL ARTS INSTRUCTION
MARTIAL WAY AND ITS VIRTUES
MASK OF THE KING
MEDITATIONS ON VIOLENCE
MERIDIAN QIGONG EXERCISES
MIND/BODY FITNESS
THE MIND INSIDE TAI CHI
THE MIND INSIDE YANG STYLE TAI CHI CHUAN
MUGAI RYU
NATURAL HEALING WITH QIGONG
NORTHERN SHAOLIN SWORD, 2ND ED.
OKINAWA'S COMPLETE KARATE SYSTEM: ISSHIN RYU
POWER BODY
PRINCIPLES OF TRADITIONAL CHINESE MEDICINE
QIGONG FOR HEALTH & MARTIAL ARTS 2ND ED.

QIGONG FOR LIVING
QIGONG FOR TREATING COMMON AILMENTS
QIGONG MASSAGE
QIGONG MEDITATION: EMBRYONIC BREATHING
QIGONG MEDITATION: SMALL CIRCULATION
QIGONG, THE SECRET OF YOUTH: DA MO'S CLASSICS
QUIET TEACHER: A XENON PEARL MARTIAL ARTS THRILLER
RAVEN'S WARRIOR
REDEMPTION
ROOT OF CHINESE QIGONG, 2ND ED.
SCALING FORCE
SENSEI: A CONNOR BURKE MARTIAL ARTS THRILLER
SHIHAN TE: THE BUNKAI OF KATA
SHIN GI TAI: KARATE TRAINING FOR BODY, MIND, AND SPIRIT
SIMPLE CHINESE MEDICINE
SIMPLE QIGONG EXERCISES FOR HEALTH, 3RD ED.
SIMPLIFIED TAI CHI CHUAN, 2ND ED.
SIMPLIFIED TAI CHI FOR BEGINNERS
SOLO TRAINING
SOLO TRAINING 2
SUDDEN DAWN: THE EPIC JOURNEY OF BODHIDHARMA
SUMO FOR MIXED MARTIAL ARTS
SUNRISE TAI CHI
SUNSET TAI CHI
SURVIVING ARMED ASSAULTS
TAE KWON DO: THE KOREAN MARTIAL ART
TAEKWONDO BLACK BELT POOMSAE
TAEKWONDO: A PATH TO EXCELLENCE
TAEKWONDO: ANCIENT WISDOM FOR THE MODERN
    WARRIOR
TAEKWONDO: DEFENSES AGAINST WEAPONS
TAEKWONDO: SPIRIT AND PRACTICE
TAO OF BIOENERGETICS
TAI CHI BALL QIGONG: FOR HEALTH AND MARTIAL ARTS
TAI CHI BALL WORKOUT FOR BEGINNERS
TAI CHI BOOK
TAI CHI CHIN NA: THE SEIZING ART OF TAI CHI CHUAN, 2ND
    ED.
TAI CHI CHUAN CLASSICAL YANG STYLE, 2ND ED.
TAI CHI CHUAN MARTIAL APPLICATIONS
TAI CHI CHUAN MARTIAL POWER, 3RD ED.
TAI CHI CONNECTIONS
TAI CHI DYNAMICS
TAI CHI FOR DEPRESSION
TAI CHI IN 10 WEEKS
TAI CHI QIGONG, 3RD ED.
TAI CHI SECRETS OF THE ANCIENT MASTERS
TAI CHI SECRETS OF THE WU & LI STYLES
TAI CHI SECRETS OF THE WU STYLE
TAI CHI SECRETS OF THE YANG STYLE
TAI CHI SWORD: CLASSICAL YANG STYLE, 2ND ED.
TAI CHI SWORD FOR BEGINNERS
TAI CHI WALKING
TAIJIQUAN THEORY OF DR. YANG, JWING-MING
TENGU: THE MOUNTAIN GOBLIN, A CONNOR BURKE
    MARTIAL ARTS THRILLER
TIMING IN THE FIGHTING ARTS
TRADITIONAL CHINESE HEALTH SECRETS
TRADITIONAL TAEKWONDO
TRAINING FOR SUDDEN VIOLENCE
WAY OF KATA
WAY OF KENDO AND KENJITSU
WAY OF SANCHIN KATA
WAY TO BLACK BELT
WESTERN HERBS FOR MARTIAL ARTISTS
WILD GOOSE QIGONG
WOMAN'S QIGONG GUIDE
XINGYIQUAN

DVDS FROM YMAA

more products available from . . .
YMAA Publication Center, Inc. 楊氏東方文化出版中心
1-800-669-8892 • info@ymaa.com • www.ymaa.com